14-DAY GREEN SMOOTHIE CLEANSE CHALLENGE

The Proven Way to Purify Your Body, Burn Worthless Fats and Lose Weight with Ease

NATALIE KENT

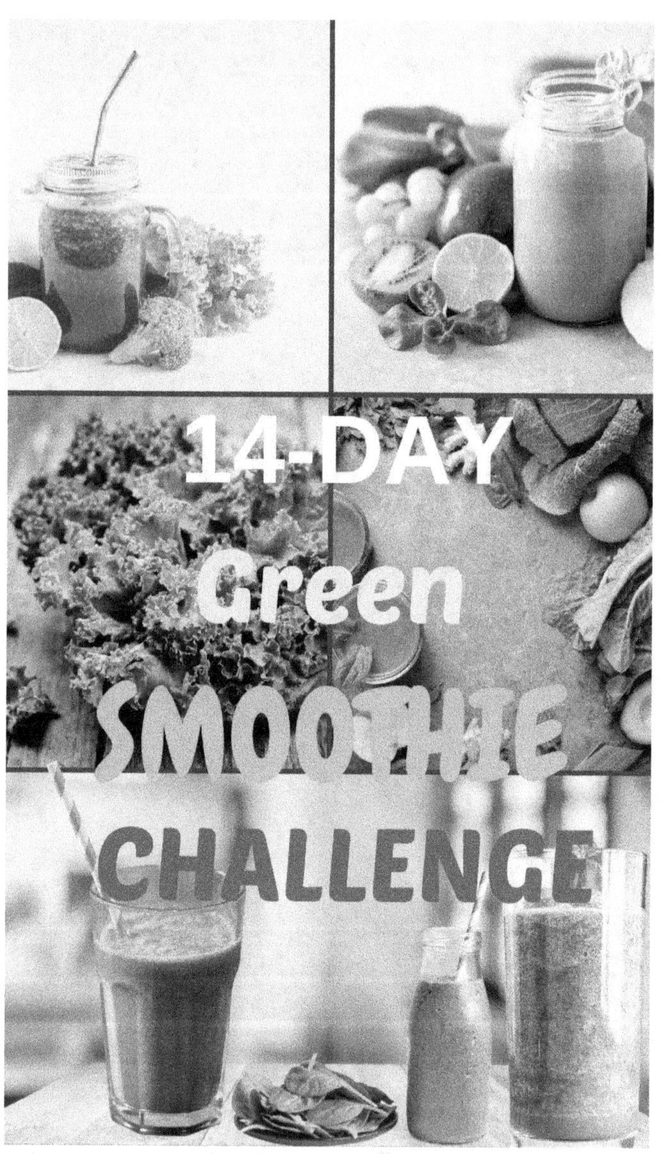
14-DAY
Green
SMOOTHIE
CHALLENGE

Contents

This page was intentionally left blank.

Chapter 1: Understanding the 14-Day Green Smoothie Cleanse Challenge

What Makes This Cleanse Unique and Effective?

Emily and I were more than just neighbors in the sunny city of Miami; we were kindred spirits, united by our shared love for health and vitality. Back then, Emily possessed a figure that turned heads—a graceful hourglass silhouette that seemed to effortlessly navigate the world around her. But life has a way of throwing unexpected curves, and as time passed, our lives took divergent paths.

Years later, fate intervened in the form of a friend request on Facebook, reigniting a friendship that had faded into the recesses of memory. It was during one of our virtual catch-ups that I shared with Emily the transformative power of green smoothies—a revelation that would forever alter the trajectory of her health and wellness journey.

As Emily navigated the joys and challenges of motherhood, her once-toned physique gradually succumbed to the pressures of postpartum life. Yet, amidst the sleepless nights and endless diaper changes, she remained determined to reclaim her vitality and zest for life.

Armed with little more than a blender and a handful of fresh ingredients, Emily embarked on a journey of self-discovery, embracing the vibrant world of green smoothies with unwavering determination. What followed was nothing short of remarkable—a metamorphosis that transcended the physical realm and touched the very core of her being.

With each sip of her morning smoothie, Emily felt a surge of energy coursing through her veins, invigorating her body and lifting her spirits. The excess weight that had stubbornly clung to her frame began to melt away, revealing the radiant beauty that had always resided within.

But it wasn't just the outward transformations that left me in awe; it was the profound shift in

Emily's mindset and outlook on life. With each passing day, she radiated a newfound sense of confidence and vitality, inspiring all who crossed her path.

As I witnessed Emily's journey unfold, I couldn't help but marvel at the transformative power of the 14-Day Green Smoothie Challenge. It wasn't merely about shedding pounds or fitting into a smaller dress size; it was about reclaiming control of one's health, rediscovering the joy of nourishing oneself from the inside out, and embracing the boundless potential that lies within each and every one of us.

So, what exactly makes this cleanse unique and effective? In essence, it is the perfect marriage of simplicity and efficacy—a potent blend of nutrient-dense greens, luscious fruits, and healing superfoods, meticulously crafted to nourish and revitalize the body from the inside out.

But beyond the ingredients themselves, it is the holistic approach of the 14-Day Green Smoothie Challenge that sets it apart. By embracing the principles of whole foods nutrition, mindful eating, and self-care, this cleanse transcends the realm of mere weight loss or detoxification, offering a pathway to true transformation and lifelong wellness.

Do You Need to Detox/Cleanse?

Take this quiz to assess whether you may benefit from a detoxification and cleansing program to eliminate toxins from your body and improve your overall health.

Read each question carefully and give yourself one point for every "yes" answer.

- ☐ Do you frequently feel sad or depressed?
- ☐ Do you often feel anxious, antsy, or stressed?
- ☐ Do you experience acne, breakouts, rashes, or hives?
- ☐ Do you have less than one bowel movement per day or experience occasional constipation?
- ☐ Do you struggle with insomnia or have trouble getting restful sleep?
- ☐ Do you experience blurred vision or itchy, burning eyes?

- [ ] Do you regularly crave sugary foods like sweets, bread, pasta, white rice, and/or potatoes?
- [ ] Do you consume processed foods (e.g., TV dinners, lunch meats, bacon, canned soup, snack bars) or fast foods at least three times a week?
- [ ] Do you drink caffeinated beverages like coffee and tea more than twice daily?
- [ ] Do you consume diet sodas or use artificial sweeteners at least once a day?
- [ ] Do you sleep less than eight hours per day?
- [ ] Do you drink less than 64 ounces of water daily?
- [ ] Are you highly sensitive to smoke, chemicals, or environmental fumes?
- [ ] Have you ever taken antibiotics, antidepressants, or other medications?
- [ ] Have you ever taken birth control pills or other estrogen-based medications?
- [ ] Do you experience frequent yeast infections?
- [ ] Do you have dental fillings containing mercury ("silver" fillings)?

- ☐ Do you regularly use commercial household cleaners, cosmetics, or deodorants?
- ☐ Do you consume non-organic vegetables, fruits, or meat?
- ☐ Have you ever smoked or been exposed to secondhand smoke?
- ☐ Are you overweight or do you have cellulite/fatty deposits?
- ☐ Does your occupation expose you to environmental toxins?
- ☐ Do you live in a major metropolitan area or near a large airport?
- ☐ Do you frequently feel tired, fatigued, or sluggish throughout the day?
- ☐ Do you have difficulty concentrating or focusing?
- ☐ Do you experience bloating, indigestion, or frequent gas after eating?
- ☐ Do you suffer from more than two colds or cases of the flu per year?
- ☐ Do you have recurring congestion, sinus issues, or postnasal drip?
- ☐ Do you notice bad breath, a coated tongue, or strong-smelling urine?
- ☐ Do you have puffy eyes or dark circles under your eyes?

Scoring:
- 20 or higher: You may significantly benefit from a detoxification program to eliminate toxins and improve your health and vitality.
- 5 to 19: You may benefit from a detoxification program for improved health and vitality.
- Below 5: You may have minimal toxic overload in your body and may already be living a healthy, toxin-free life.

Remember, the accumulation of toxins in the body can lead to various health issues, including weight gain and fatigue. The 14-Day Green Smoothie Cleanse offers a transformative experience to detoxify your body and improve your overall well-being.

Here's how to do it:

1. Drink up to 60 ounces of green smoothies daily, divided into thirds and consumed throughout the day.

2. Snack on crunchy vegetables like apples, celery, carrots, and cucumbers, or high-protein snacks such as unsweetened peanut butter,

hard-boiled eggs, and raw or unsalted nuts and seeds.

3. Stay hydrated by drinking at least eight glasses of water (64 ounces) per day, along with detox or herbal teas as desired.

4. Perform one of the two methods for colon cleansing as needed.

5. Avoid consuming refined sugar, meat, dairy, alcohol, coffee, soda, processed foods, fried foods, and refined carbohydrates during the cleanse.

Committing to the 14-Day Green Smoothie Cleanse can jumpstart your journey to improved health and vitality by eliminating toxins from your body and restoring balance to your system.

In the pages that follow, we will delve deep into the core principles of the 14-Day Green Smoothie Cleanse Challenge, exploring the science behind its efficacy, unraveling the mysteries of its transformative power, and equipping you with the tools and knowledge you need to embark on your own journey of health and healing.

So, are you ready to embark on the adventure of a lifetime? Are you ready to unlock the boundless potential that lies within you? If so, then join up as we embark on the 14-Day Green Smoothie Challenge—a journey that promises not only to rejuvenate your body but to nourish your soul and awaken your spirit.

Chapter 2: Why Should it be Green Smoothies?

Exploring the Power of Green Nutrition

In the vast array of dietary trends and wellness fads, one simple yet powerful concoction stands out amidst the noise—the green smoothie. Green smoothies have emerged as a powerhouse in the realm of health and wellness, rapidly gaining popularity for their simplicity and profound nutritional benefits. Comprised of raw organic fruits, leafy greens, and water, these vibrant blends offer a whole load of advantages that contribute to a healthier lifestyle.

But what exactly makes this vibrant blend of leafy greens and fresh fruits so special? Join me as we unravel the mysteries of green nutrition and discover why green smoothies have become the cornerstone of countless health journeys around the world.

The allure of green smoothies lies in their simplicity and versatility. At their core, green smoothies are a potent blend of leafy greens—such as spinach, kale, or Swiss chard—and fruits—such as bananas, berries, or apples—combined with liquid, such as water, coconut water, or almond milk. But don't let their humble ingredients fool you; within these vibrant concoctions lies a powerhouse of nutrients and healing compounds that can nourish and revitalize the body from the inside out.

One of the primary reasons why green smoothies have gained such widespread popularity is their unparalleled nutrient density. Leafy greens, in particular, are packed with essential vitamins, minerals, and antioxidants that are crucial for optimal health and vitality. From vitamin C and vitamin K to folate and iron, these nutrient-rich greens provide a veritable cornucopia of essential nutrients that support everything from immune function to cardiovascular health.

But perhaps the most remarkable aspect of green smoothies is their ability to harness the potent healing power of chlorophyll.

Responsible for giving plants their vibrant green hue, chlorophyll is a powerhouse nutrient that boasts a myriad of health benefits. Not only does chlorophyll help to oxygenate the blood and alkalize the body, but it also acts as a powerful detoxifier, helping to rid the body of harmful toxins and impurities.

Another compelling reason to embrace green smoothies is their role in promoting optimal digestion and gut health. Thanks to their high fiber content, green smoothies help to support healthy digestion, regulate bowel movements, and promote the growth of beneficial gut bacteria. This not only aids in nutrient absorption but also helps to alleviate common digestive complaints such as bloating, gas, and constipation.

But perhaps the most compelling reason to incorporate green smoothies into your daily routine is their unrivaled ability to support weight management and promote overall wellness. By providing a convenient and delicious way to increase your intake of nutrient-dense fruits and vegetables, green smoothies can help to curb cravings, boost metabolism, and promote satiety, making it easier to maintain a healthy weight and lifestyle.

In addition to their physical health benefits, green smoothies also offer a myriad of mental and emotional benefits. From increased energy and mental clarity to enhanced mood and focus, the nutrient-rich blend of greens and fruits can help to nourish not only the body but also the mind and spirit.

But perhaps the most compelling reason to embrace green smoothies is the profound impact they can have on your overall quality of life. By nourishing your body with the vital nutrients it needs to thrive, green smoothies can help you to feel more vibrant, energized, and alive than ever before. Whether you're looking to lose weight, boost your energy levels, or simply enhance your overall well-being, green smoothies offer a simple yet powerful solution that can help you achieve your health goals and live your best life.

So, why choose green smoothies? In essence, they offer a convenient, delicious, and incredibly effective way to nourish your body with the vital nutrients it needs to thrive. From supporting digestion and gut health to promoting weight management and overall wellness, green smoothies offer a myriad of benefits that can help you look and feel your best from the inside out.

In retrospect, here are ten compelling reasons to incorporate green smoothies into your daily routine:

1. Detoxification: Our bodies are constantly exposed to toxins from various sources, which can impede the natural detoxification processes. Green smoothies offer a gentle yet effective way to support detoxification and eliminate harmful substances that can hinder health and contribute to weight gain. By supplying essential nutrients and fiber, green smoothies aid in cleansing the digestive system and promoting toxin elimination.

2. Weight Loss: If you're aiming to shed excess weight, green smoothies are an invaluable ally. With their high water content and abundance of green vegetables, they provide satiety without excess calories. Furthermore, the fiber-rich nature of green smoothies helps curb cravings and promote feelings of fullness,

making weight loss more attainable and sustainable.

3. Vibrant, Radiant Health: Optimal health radiates from within, manifesting as boundless energy and vitality. Embracing a diet rich in natural, raw foods nourishes the body at the cellular level, promoting a vibrant and youthful appearance. As you fuel your body with clean, nutrient-dense ingredients, you'll notice improvements in both your physical well-being and your overall complexion.

4. Nutrient-Rich: Green smoothies are bursting with essential nutrients, including vitamins, minerals, antioxidants, and phytonutrients. Unlike cooked foods, which can lose nutrients due to high temperatures, the raw ingredients in green smoothies retain their nutritional integrity. Additionally, the chlorophyll found in leafy greens closely resembles human blood, offering a cleansing and rejuvenating effect akin to a natural blood transfusion.

5. Increased Energy Levels: Green smoothies provide a potent source of natural energy, thanks to their nutrient-rich composition. Unlike caffeine or sugar-laden beverages, which offer

temporary spikes followed by crashes, green smoothies deliver sustained energy throughout the day. By nourishing your body with wholesome ingredients, you'll experience enhanced vitality and stamina to tackle daily challenges.

6. Enhanced Digestive Health: A healthy digestive system is essential for overall well-being, and green smoothies play a key role in supporting digestive health. The fiber content in green smoothies promotes regularity and helps prevent digestive issues such as bloating and constipation. Additionally, the enzymes present in raw fruits and vegetables aid in digestion, ensuring optimal nutrient absorption and gut function.

7. Improved Hydration: Proper hydration is fundamental for numerous bodily functions, yet many people struggle to meet their daily water intake requirements. Green smoothies offer a delicious and hydrating alternative to plain water, helping you stay adequately hydrated throughout the day. By incorporating hydrating fruits and vegetables into your smoothies, you'll support optimal cellular function and maintain overall hydration levels.

8. Antioxidant Protection: Antioxidants play a crucial role in defending the body against oxidative stress and free radical damage, which can contribute to chronic disease and premature aging. Green smoothies are rich in antioxidants from ingredients such as berries, leafy greens, and citrus fruits, providing potent protection against cellular damage and inflammation.

9. Alkalizing Properties: Maintaining a slightly alkaline pH balance in the body is essential for optimal health and vitality. Many processed foods and unhealthy dietary habits can lead to excess acidity, which can disrupt bodily functions and contribute to inflammation and disease. Green smoothies, with their alkalizing properties, help restore balance and promote a more alkaline environment within the body.

10. Convenient and Versatile: Incorporating green smoothies into your daily routine is both convenient and versatile. With endless flavor combinations and the ability to customize ingredients based on personal preferences, green smoothies offer a flexible and enjoyable way to boost your nutrient intake. Whether

enjoyed as a meal replacement, snack, or post-workout refresher, green smoothies provide a convenient solution for busy lifestyles.

By embracing green smoothies as a regular part of your dietary regimen, you'll reap a multitude of benefits that contribute to improved health, vitality, and overall well-being. Whether you're looking to lose weight, increase energy, or simply nourish your body with essential nutrients, green smoothies offer a delicious and effective solution for achieving your health goals.

In addition to their health benefits, green smoothies are also cost-effective, especially if you make them at home. While a vegetable smoothie at a juice bar may set you back up to $7, a homemade green smoothie may only cost you $2 – $3 on average. By shopping at your local farmer's market, you stand the chance of saving even more money while getting the freshest fruit and vegetables out there.

In the pages that follow, we will delve deeper into the science behind green smoothies, exploring the specific nutrients and compounds that make them so beneficial for health and vitality. We will also provide practical tips and strategies for incorporating green smoothies into your daily routine, ensuring that you can reap the full spectrum of benefits that these vibrant concoctions have to offer.

Chapter 3: Preparing for Success

Essential Steps to Ensure a Smooth Transition

Going on a journey towards health and wellness is an exciting endeavor, but it requires careful planning and preparation to ensure success. In this chapter, we will explore the essential steps you need to take to prepare for your 14-Day Green Smoothie Challenge. From stocking your kitchen with the necessary ingredients to mentally preparing yourself for the journey ahead, each step is crucial in laying the foundation for a smooth and successful transition.

Step 1: Set Clear Goals

Before diving into any new health regimen, it's important to define your goals and objectives. Take some time to reflect on why you're embarking on the 14-Day Green Smoothie Challenge. Are you looking to lose weight, boost your energy levels, or improve your overall health and well-being? By setting clear and specific goals, you'll have a roadmap to guide you through the challenge and keep you motivated along the way.

Step 2: Educate Yourself

Knowledge is power, and when it comes to embarking on a new dietary regimen, it's essential to educate yourself about the principles behind it. Take some time to research the benefits of green smoothies, familiarize yourself with the types of ingredients you'll be using, and learn about the potential health benefits they offer. The more you understand about the science behind green smoothies, the more motivated and empowered you'll feel to stick with the challenge.

Step 3: Stock Your Kitchen and Create a Shopping List

One of the keys to success in any dietary challenge is having the right ingredients on hand. Take inventory of your kitchen and make a list of the ingredients you'll need for your green smoothies.

Now that you're committed to the 14-Day Green Smoothie Challenge, it's time to stock your kitchen with all the essential ingredients and create a comprehensive shopping list. Here's a breakdown of what you'll need:

Produce:
- Spinach
- Kale
- Swiss chard
- Romaine lettuce
- Cucumber
- Celery
- Tiger nuts
- Carrots
- Beets
- Bell peppers (assorted colors)
- Tomatoes
- Avocado
- Zucchini
- Broccoli
- Cauliflower
- Brussels sprouts
- Green apples
- Berries (strawberries, blueberries, raspberries, blackberries)
- Pineapple
- Mango
- Kiwi
- Oranges

- Lemons
- Limes
- Bananas

Frozen Produce:
- Mixed berries
- Mixed tropical fruit blend (pineapple, mango, papaya)
- Mixed berry blend (strawberries, blueberries, raspberries)
- Sliced peaches

Herbs:
- Parsley
- Cilantro
- Mint
- Basil

Dairy and Alternatives:
- Greek yogurt
- Almond milk
- Coconut milk
- Tiger nut milk

Protein Sources:
- Chicken breast
- Turkey breast
- Lean beef (e.g., sirloin)

- Salmon fillets
- Tofu
- Tempeh
- Lentils
- Chickpeas
- Black beans

Grains and Legumes:
- Quinoa
- Brown rice
- Whole grain bread
- Whole grain pasta

Nuts and Seeds:
- Almonds
- Walnuts
- Chia seeds
- Flaxseeds
- Hemp seeds
- Pumpkin seeds

Other Pantry Staples:
- Olive oil
- Coconut oil
- Balsamic vinegar
- Honey or maple syrup
- Dijon mustard
- Garlic

- Ginger
- Turmeric
- Cinnamon
- Nutmeg
- Cumin
- Paprika
- Sea salt
- Black pepper

Miscellaneous:
- Protein powder (optional)
- Green tea bags
- Rolled oats

As you create your shopping list, be sure to take into account the number of servings you'll be making each day and adjust the quantities accordingly. It's also a good idea to check your pantry and refrigerator for any ingredients you may already have on hand to avoid unnecessary duplication.

Once you've finalized your shopping list, head to the grocery store or farmers' market to gather all your ingredients. Consider choosing organic produce whenever possible to minimize exposure to pesticides and maximize nutrient density.

By stocking your kitchen with all the necessary ingredients and creating a comprehensive shopping list, you'll be fully prepared to tackle the 14-Day Green Smoothie Challenge with confidence and ease. So grab your reusable shopping bags and get ready to embark on a journey towards better health and vitality!

Step 4: Invest in Quality Equipment
Having the right equipment can make all the difference when it comes to preparing green smoothies. Invest in a high-quality blender that can handle tough leafy greens and frozen fruits with ease. A blender with multiple speed settings and a powerful motor will ensure that your smoothies come out smooth and creamy every time.

Step 5: Plan Your Meals
To ensure that you stay on track with your 14-Day Green Smoothie Challenge, it's important to plan your meals ahead of time. Take some time each week to plan out your meals and snacks, making sure to incorporate plenty of fresh fruits and vegetables into your diet. Consider prepping some of your ingredients in advance, such as washing and

chopping your greens or pre-packaging your smoothie ingredients, to make mealtime a breeze.

Step 6: Clear Out Temptations

To set yourself up for success, it's important to remove any temptations from your kitchen that may derail your progress. Take some time to clear out any unhealthy or processed foods from your pantry and refrigerator, replacing them with wholesome, nutrient-dense options. Having a clean and clutter-free kitchen will make it easier to stick to your green smoothie challenge and resist temptation.

Step 7: Mentally Prepare Yourself

Embarking on a new dietary regimen can be challenging, both physically and mentally. Take some time to mentally prepare yourself for the journey ahead, acknowledging that there may be obstacles and challenges along the way. Practice positive self-talk and visualization techniques to help build your confidence and keep you motivated throughout the challenge.

Step 8: Establish a Support System

Having a strong support system in place can make all the difference when it comes to achieving your health and wellness goals. Reach out to friends, family members, or online communities who can offer encouragement, accountability, and support as you navigate the 14-Day Green Smoothie Challenge. Having someone to share your successes and struggles with can help keep you motivated and on track.

Step 9: Practice Self-Care
Lastly, remember to prioritize self-care throughout the 14-Day Green Smoothie Challenge. Take time each day to engage in activities that nourish your body, mind, and soul, whether it's going for a walk in nature, practicing mindfulness meditation, or indulging in a relaxing bath. Taking care of yourself holistically will help ensure that you have the energy and motivation to stick with the challenge and reap its full benefits.

By following these essential steps to prepare for success, you'll be well-equipped to embark on your 14-Day Green Smoothie Challenge with confidence and determination. Remember to stay focused on your goals, stay flexible in your approach, and most importantly, enjoy the journey towards better health and wellness.

Chapter 4: Navigating the 14-Day Green Smoothie Challenge

A Step-by-Step Guide to Your Cleanse Journey

Journeying through the 14-Day Green Smoothie Challenge is an exciting and transformative journey towards better health and vitality. In this chapter, we will provide you with a comprehensive, step-by-step guide to navigating the challenge with confidence and ease. From preparing your first green smoothie to overcoming common challenges along the way, we'll walk you through each stage of the cleanse journey to ensure that you achieve optimal results and emerge feeling rejuvenated and revitalized.

Step 1: Preparation

Before diving headfirst into the 14-Day Green Smoothie Challenge, it's essential to take some time to prepare both mentally and physically. Start by setting clear goals for yourself and envisioning the positive changes you hope to achieve during the cleanse. Take inventory of your kitchen and stock up on all the necessary ingredients, making sure to have an ample supply of leafy greens, fruits, and liquid bases on hand. Consider prepping some of your ingredients in advance to streamline the process and save time during the challenge.

Step 2: Start Slowly

As you embark on the 14-Day Green Smoothie Challenge, it's important to ease into it gradually to give your body time to adjust to the new dietary regimen. Begin by replacing one meal or snack each day with a green smoothie, gradually increasing the frequency as you feel more comfortable. This gradual approach will help minimize any potential detox symptoms and ensure a smooth transition to a healthier diet.

Step 3: Experiment with Recipes

One of the joys of the 14-Day Green Smoothie Challenge is the opportunity to experiment with a wide variety of recipes and flavor combinations. Don't be afraid to get creative and try out different combinations of leafy greens, fruits, and superfood additions to find what works best for you. Consider incorporating seasonal produce or local ingredients to add variety and freshness to your smoothies. Keep track of your favorite recipes so you can recreate them throughout the challenge.

Step 4: Stay Hydrated

Proper hydration is essential during the 14-Day Green Smoothie Challenge to support the body's natural detoxification processes and keep you feeling energized and refreshed. In addition to drinking your green smoothies, be sure to consume plenty of water throughout the day to stay hydrated. Consider adding a slice of lemon or cucumber to your water for added flavor and hydration benefits.

Step 5: Listen to Your Body

As you navigate the 14-Day Green Smoothie Challenge, it's important to listen to your body and honor its needs. Pay attention to how you feel after consuming each smoothie and adjust your ingredients or portion sizes accordingly. If you experience any discomfort or adverse reactions, such as bloating or digestive issues, take note of the ingredients you used and consider modifying your recipes in the future.

Step 6: Practice Self-Care

The process of dietary cleanse can be physically and emotionally taxing, so it's important to prioritize self-care throughout the 14-Day Green Smoothie Challenge. Take time each day to engage in activities that nourish your body, mind, and soul, whether it's going for a walk in nature, practicing yoga, or indulging in a relaxing bath. Remember to practice mindfulness and gratitude, focusing on the positive changes you're making for your health and well-being.

Step 7: Stay Flexible

While the 14-Day Green Smoothie Challenge provides a structured framework for cleansing and rejuvenation, it's important to stay flexible and adapt to the needs of your body. If you find that certain ingredients or recipes don't agree with you, don't be afraid to switch things up and try something new. Listen to your intuition and trust that your body knows what it needs to thrive.

Step 8: Celebrate Your Successes

As you near the end of the 14-Day Green Smoothie Challenge, take some time to reflect on your accomplishments and celebrate how far you've come. Whether you've experienced weight loss, increased energy, or improved digestion, each success is a testament to your dedication and commitment to your health and well-being. Treat yourself to a special reward or indulge in a healthy treat to commemorate your achievements and motivate you to continue on your journey towards optimal health.

By following this step-by-step guide to navigating the 14-Day Green Smoothie Challenge, you'll be well-equipped to embark on your cleanse journey with confidence and ease. Remember to stay focused on your goals, stay flexible in your approach, and most importantly, enjoy the journey towards better health and vitality. With each green smoothie you sip, you'll be one step closer to unlocking the vibrant, energized version of yourself that lies within.

Preparation for Nutrient-Enriched Smoothies

Before embarking on your 14-Day Green Smoothie Cleanse journey, it's vital to ensure that your ingredients are thoroughly cleaned and prepared to unlock their full nutritional potential. Follow these essential steps to wash and prep your ingredients before blending your refreshing and nourishing smoothies:

1. Thoroughly Clean Fresh Produce: Start by rinsing all fruits and vegetables under cool or warm running water, even if you plan to peel them later. This initial step helps eliminate any surface impurities, pesticides, or residues, ensuring that you extract the maximum nutrients from your ingredients.

2. Peel and Remove Cores as Needed: For fruits with thick skins or inedible cores, such as mangoes, kiwis, pineapples, and papayas, it's essential to peel and core them before use. Removing these parts ensures a smoother texture and enhances the overall taste of your smoothies.

3. Cut into Bite-Sized Pieces: To facilitate the blending process and achieve a silky-smooth consistency, chop larger fruits and vegetables into smaller, bite-sized pieces. This preparatory step ensures that your blender can effortlessly blend all ingredients, resulting in a velvety-smooth blend and also prolong the life of your blender.

4. Pre-Soak Chia Seeds: If your recipes include chia seeds, consider soaking them in water for a few minutes before blending. This simple pre-soaking technique helps soften the seeds and improves their texture, allowing your body to absorb their valuable nutrients more efficiently.

5. Select Fresh, High-Quality Ingredients: Opt for fresh, top-quality ingredients to elevate the nutritional value and flavor profile of your 14-Day Green Smoothie Cleanse. Fresh produce not only enhances the taste but also guarantees that you receive the highest concentration of essential nutrients.

By following these straightforward yet crucial preparation guidelines, you'll lay the foundation for crafting nutrient-packed and revitalizing smoothies throughout your cleanse, leaving you feeling invigorated and nourished.

Chapter 5: Insider Tips for Ease and Maximum Results

Expert Advice and Strategies for Success

New to green smoothies and finding it hard to adjust to the green color? Start by incorporating baby spinach into your smoothies. Baby spinach has a mild flavor and blends well with fruits, making it a perfect choice for beginners. You'll reap the nutritional benefits without noticing the taste of the greens. As you become accustomed to green smoothies, gradually increase the greens and experiment with different varieties like kale or chard for added variety and nutrients.

In this chapter, we'll delve into advanced tips and expert advice to help you optimize your cleanse experience and achieve outstanding results. These insider strategies will elevate your cleanse journey, enabling you to harness the full potential of green smoothies for improved health and vitality.

Tip 1: Experiment with Greens

While spinach and kale are popular choices for green smoothies, don't be afraid to experiment with a variety of leafy greens to diversify your nutrient intake. Try incorporating lesser-known greens such as collard greens, Swiss chard, or beet greens into your smoothies for unique flavors and added health benefits. Each type of green offers its own unique combination of vitamins, minerals, and antioxidants, so mix it up to maximize your nutrient intake and keep your taste buds engaged.

Tip 2: Balance Your Smoothies

Achieving the perfect balance of flavors, textures, and nutrients is key to creating delicious and satisfying green smoothies. Aim to include a mix of fruits, vegetables, and healthy fats in each smoothie to ensure a well-rounded nutritional profile. Consider adding avocado, coconut oil, or nut butter to your smoothies for added creaminess and satiety. Experiment with different flavor combinations to find what works best for you, and don't be afraid to get creative with your ingredients.

Tip 3: Enhance with Herbs and Spices

Herbs and spices are powerful flavor enhancers that can take your green smoothies to the next level. Experiment with adding fresh herbs such as mint, basil, or cilantro to your smoothies for a burst of freshness and complexity. Incorporate spices like cinnamon, ginger, or turmeric for added warmth and depth of flavor. Not only do herbs and spices enhance the taste of your smoothies, but they also offer a wide range of health benefits, from reducing inflammation to supporting digestion.

Tip 4: Boost with Protein

Adding protein to your green smoothies is a great way to increase satiety, support muscle repair and growth, and stabilize blood sugar levels. Consider incorporating protein-rich ingredients such as Greek yogurt, silken tofu, or plant-based protein powder into your smoothies for an added nutritional boost. Protein-packed smoothies are especially beneficial for post-workout recovery or as a satisfying meal replacement option during your cleanse.

Tip 5: Practice Food Combining

Food combining is a dietary principle that involves pairing foods together in a way that optimizes digestion and nutrient absorption. While green smoothies are inherently well-balanced in terms of macronutrients, you can further enhance their digestibility by paying attention to food combining principles. For example, avoid combining high-protein foods with high-carbohydrate foods in the same smoothie, as this can lead to digestive discomfort. Instead, focus on combining greens with fruits and healthy fats for optimal digestion and nutrient assimilation.

Tip 6: Listen to Your Cravings

As you progress through the 14-Day Green Smoothie Challenge, pay attention to any cravings or food preferences that arise. Cravings can be a powerful indicator of your body's nutritional needs, so listen to them and adjust your smoothie recipes accordingly. If you find yourself craving sweets, experiment with adding naturally sweet fruits like bananas or dates to your smoothies. If you're craving something savory, try incorporating ingredients like avocado or cucumber for a more satisfying flavor profile.

Tip 7: Support Your Gut Health

Gut health plays a crucial role in overall health and well-being, so it's important to support your digestive system during your cleanse journey. Consider adding gut-friendly ingredients such as probiotic-rich yogurt, fermented foods like kefir or kimchi, and prebiotic-rich foods like garlic or onions to your smoothies to promote a healthy balance of gut bacteria. Supporting your gut health will not only enhance digestion but also strengthen your immune system and improve nutrient absorption.

Tip 8: Practice Gratitude and Mindfulness

Cleansing is not just about nourishing your body with healthy foods; it's also about cultivating a positive mindset and fostering a sense of gratitude and mindfulness. Take time each day to express gratitude for the nourishing foods you're consuming and the positive changes you're experiencing in your health and well-being. Practice mindfulness during meal times, focusing on the sensory experience of eating and savoring each bite. Cultivating a mindset of gratitude and mindfulness will enhance your cleanse experience and support your overall health and vitality.

By incorporating these advanced tips and expert strategies into your cleanse journey, you'll elevate your green smoothie experience to new heights and achieve maximum results. Remember to stay open-minded, embrace experimentation, and trust in the transformative power of green nutrition. With each sip of your green smoothie, you're nourishing your body, mind, and soul, and taking an important step towards vibrant health and vitality.

Chapter 6: Sustaining Your Progress Beyond the Cleanse

Building on Your Achievements for Long-Term Wellness

As you reflect on the completion of your 14-Day Green Smoothie Cleanse, it's time to shift focus towards maintaining your progress for sustained wellness. This chapter explores strategies and techniques to build upon your cleanse experience, fostering habits that support long-term health and vitality.

Reflecting on Your Cleanse Journey

Before we delve into sustaining your progress, take a moment to reflect on your cleanse journey. Consider the physical, mental, and emotional changes you've experienced over the past 14 days. Did you notice improvements in energy levels, digestion, or mood? Reflecting on these changes provides valuable insights and motivation for the next phase of your wellness journey.

Setting Sustainable Goals

Moving forward, set realistic and sustainable goals aligned with your long-term health objectives. Look beyond short-term outcomes and focus on broader goals such as improving sleep quality, increasing physical activity levels, or incorporating more whole foods into your diet. By setting achievable goals, you create a roadmap for long-term success and motivation.

Embracing a Whole Foods Diet

Adopting a whole foods-based diet is essential for sustaining progress beyond the cleanse. Whole foods, including fruits, vegetables, whole grains, nuts, seeds, and legumes, provide essential nutrients without the additives found in processed foods. Prioritize whole foods to nourish your body with vitamins, minerals, and antioxidants necessary for optimal health.

Mindful Eating Practices

Incorporate mindful eating practices into your daily routine to support long-term wellness. Pay attention to the sensory experience of eating, including taste, texture, and aroma, and listen to your body's hunger and satiety cues. By practicing mindfulness during meals, you foster a deeper connection with your food and improve digestion.

Regular Physical Activity

Regular exercise is fundamental for sustaining progress and supporting overall well-being. Choose activities you enjoy, such as walking, jogging, yoga, or strength training, and incorporate them into your daily routine. Physical activity not only benefits physical health but also reduces stress and improves mood. Whether it's through cardiovascular exercise, strength training, or yoga, aim to break a sweat regularly to support the detoxification process and maintain a healthy weight. Engage in regular exercise to promote sweating, which is one of the body's natural mechanisms for eliminating toxins.

Prioritizing Sleep and Stress Management

Quality sleep and stress management are crucial for long-term wellness. Aim for seven to nine hours of sleep each night and incorporate stress-reducing activities such as meditation, deep breathing, or spending time in nature. Prioritize self-care practices to support optimal physical and mental health.

Staying Hydrated

Hydration is essential for every aspect of health, from digestion to energy production. Drink plenty of water and herbal teas throughout the day to maintain hydration levels. Incorporate hydrating foods such as fruits and vegetables into your diet to support overall hydration.

Community Support and Accountability

Build a support network of friends, family, or like-minded individuals to sustain progress. Seek community support through online forums, social media groups, or local wellness meetups. Surround yourself with individuals who share your health goals and provide encouragement and accountability.

Flexibility and Adaptability

Approach your wellness journey with flexibility and adaptability. Life is full of unexpected challenges, and it's essential to adjust your goals and strategies accordingly. Embrace setbacks as learning experiences and remain committed to your long-term health and well-being.

Sustaining progress beyond the cleanse requires cultivating habits and practices that support long-term health and vitality. By setting sustainable goals, embracing a whole foods diet, practicing mindful eating, prioritizing physical activity, sleep, and stress management, staying hydrated, seeking community support, and maintaining flexibility and adaptability, you lay the foundation for lifelong wellness. Remember that wellness is a journey, and every step you take towards prioritizing your health is a step towards a vibrant and fulfilling life.

As you progress through the 14-Day Green Smoothie Cleanse and focus on sustaining your weight loss journey, it's crucial to explore supplementary detox methods to enhance your efforts. Let's even go deeper into various techniques and practices designed to amplify the benefits of the cleanse and support long-term weight management.

Understanding the Continuum of Detoxification

Before we go into supplementary detox methods, let's first understand the continuum of detoxification. Detoxification is not a one-time event but rather an ongoing process that occurs naturally within the body. While the 14-Day Green Smoothie Cleanse serves as a powerful catalyst for detoxification, incorporating additional methods can further support the body's ability to eliminate toxins and promote sustainable weight loss.

Hydration and Water Fasting

One of the simplest yet most effective detox methods is staying hydrated through water fasting. Water fasting involves consuming only water for a specified period, allowing the body to flush out toxins and reset its systems. While prolonged water fasting may not be suitable for everyone, short-term fasting or intermittent fasting can be incorporated into your routine to promote detoxification and support weight loss.

Intermittent Fasting

Intermittent fasting is a popular dietary approach that alternates between periods of eating and fasting. By restricting the window of time during which you consume food, intermittent fasting can enhance fat burning, improve insulin sensitivity, and promote cellular repair. Consider incorporating intermittent fasting into your post-cleanse routine to maintain the momentum of weight loss and support ongoing detoxification.

Nutrient-Dense Whole Foods

In addition to fasting, focusing on nutrient-dense whole foods is essential for sustaining weight loss and promoting detoxification. Emphasize fruits, vegetables, lean proteins, and healthy fats in your diet to provide your body with the essential nutrients it needs to thrive. By fueling your body with wholesome ingredients, you'll support optimal detoxification and maintain a healthy weight over the long term.

Incorporating Herbal Supplements

Herbal supplements can serve as valuable allies in supporting detoxification and promoting weight loss. Consider incorporating herbs such as dandelion root, milk thistle, and turmeric into your daily routine to support liver function, enhance digestion, and reduce inflammation. Be sure to consult with a healthcare professional before starting any new supplement regimen to ensure safety and effectiveness.

Sauna Therapy

Sauna therapy is another effective method for promoting detoxification and supporting weight loss. Spending time in a sauna helps increase circulation, promote sweating, and facilitate the elimination of toxins through the skin. Incorporate regular sauna sessions into your wellness routine to enhance the benefits of the cleanse and support long-term weight management.

Mind-Body Practices

In addition to physical detoxification methods, don't overlook the importance of mind-body practices in supporting weight loss and overall well-being. Techniques such as meditation, deep breathing, and mindfulness can help reduce stress, improve sleep quality, and enhance overall resilience. By cultivating a calm and balanced mind, you'll support the body's natural detoxification processes and maintain a healthy weight over time.

Consistency and Commitment

Ultimately, sustaining weight loss and promoting detoxification require consistency and commitment to healthy lifestyle habits.

While the 14-Day Green Smoothie Cleanse serves as a powerful kickstart, it's essential to maintain the momentum by incorporating ongoing detox methods into your daily routine. By prioritizing hydration, nutrient-dense foods, physical activity, and mind-body practices, you'll create a foundation for sustainable weight loss and long-term wellness.

Enhancing your cleanse with supplementary detox methods is key to sustaining weight loss and promoting optimal health over the long term. By incorporating hydration, fasting, nutrient-dense foods, herbal supplements, physical activity, sauna therapy, and mind-body practices into your routine, you'll amplify the benefits of the cleanse and support ongoing detoxification. Remember, consistency and commitment are essential for achieving lasting results, so stay focused on your goals and embrace the journey towards vibrant health and well-being.

Chapter 7: Answering Your Burning Questions

Let's address some of the most common questions and provide clear, concise answers to help alleviate any uncertainties you may have.

1. What exactly is the 14-Day Green Smoothie Cleanse?

- The 14-Day Green Smoothie Cleanse is a dietary program designed to detoxify the body, promote weight loss, and improve overall health by consuming nutrient-rich green smoothies for a period of two weeks.

2. Are green smoothies suitable for everyone?

- While green smoothies are generally considered safe for most people, it's essential to consult with a healthcare professional before starting any new dietary regimen, especially if you have underlying health conditions or dietary restrictions.

3. Do I need a blender to participate in the cleanse?

- Yes, a high-speed blender is necessary to properly blend the ingredients for green smoothies. If you don't have a blender, consider borrowing one from a friend or investing in an affordable model to ensure you can fully participate in the cleanse.

4. Can I customize the green smoothie recipes to suit my taste preferences?

- Absolutely! Feel free to experiment with different combinations of fruits, leafy greens, and other ingredients to create green smoothies that appeal to your taste buds. The key is to maintain the recommended fruit-to-greens ratio of 6:4 for optimal flavor and nutrition.

5. Will I experience any side effects during the cleanse?

- Some individuals may experience mild side effects such as headaches, fatigue, or digestive issues as the body adjusts to the cleanse. These symptoms are usually temporary and should subside as you continue with the program.

6. Can I exercise while on the cleanse?

- Yes, moderate exercise is encouraged during the cleanse to support overall health and well-being. However, listen to your body and adjust your activity level as needed, especially if you're experiencing fatigue or other symptoms.

7. Will I lose weight on the cleanse?

- While weight loss results may vary from person to person, many participants experience significant weight loss during the 14-Day Green Smoothie Cleanse, particularly if they adhere to the program guidelines and maintain a healthy lifestyle.

8. What should I do if I feel hungry between meals?

- If you feel hungry between meals, reach for healthy, whole food snacks such as fruits, vegetables, nuts, or seeds to keep you satisfied and energized throughout the day.

9. Can I drink other beverages besides green smoothies during the cleanse?

- While green smoothies should be the primary beverage during the cleanse, you can also consume water, herbal teas, and coconut water to stay hydrated and support detoxification.

10. Will I experience cravings for unhealthy foods while on the cleanse?

- It's possible to experience cravings for unhealthy foods, especially in the initial stages of the cleanse. However, as your body adjusts to the nutrient-rich green smoothies, cravings for unhealthy foods often diminish.

11. Can I consume alcohol while on the cleanse?

- Alcohol should be avoided during the cleanse, as it can interfere with the detoxification process and hinder weight loss efforts. Focus on hydrating, nourishing beverages such as water and herbal teas instead.

12. What should I do if I experience digestive discomfort during the cleanse?

- If you experience digestive discomfort such as bloating or gas, try drinking plenty of water, incorporating probiotic-rich foods into your diet, and avoiding foods that may exacerbate symptoms.

13. Will I experience increased energy levels while on the cleanse?

   - Many participants report increased energy levels and improved vitality as they progress through the cleanse. However, individual results may vary, so listen to your body and adjust your activity level accordingly.

14. Can I continue taking my regular medications and supplements while on the cleanse?

   - It's important to continue taking any prescribed medications as directed by your healthcare provider. However, if you have concerns about specific supplements, consult with a healthcare professional for guidance.

15. Is it safe to do the cleanse while pregnant or breastfeeding?

   - Pregnant and breastfeeding women should avoid undertaking the cleanse due to the potential impact on nutrient intake and overall health. It's crucial to prioritize the nutritional needs of both mother and baby during this time.

16. Can I do the cleanse if I have a medical condition such as diabetes or high blood pressure?

- Individuals with medical conditions should consult with a healthcare professional before starting the cleanse to ensure it is safe and appropriate for their individual needs.

17. Will I experience detox symptoms such as headaches or fatigue?

- Some participants may experience mild detox symptoms such as headaches, fatigue, or irritability as the body eliminates toxins. These symptoms are usually temporary and indicate that the cleanse is working.

18. Can I consume caffeine while on the cleanse?

- It's best to avoid caffeine during the cleanse, as it can interfere with the detoxification process and disrupt sleep patterns. Opt for caffeine-free beverages like herbal teas or water instead.

19. What should I do if I experience intense hunger or cravings during the cleanse?

- If you experience intense hunger or cravings, try increasing your intake of green smoothies and whole food snacks to keep you satisfied. Additionally, practicing mindfulness techniques such as deep breathing or meditation can help curb cravings.

20. Can I do the cleanse if I have a nut allergy?

- If you have a nut allergy, you can customize the green smoothie recipes to exclude nuts or substitute them with seeds or seed butter. Be sure to read ingredient labels carefully and avoid any allergens.

21. Will I experience changes in my bowel movements during the cleanse?

- It's common to experience changes in bowel movements during the cleanse as the body eliminates toxins and waste products. However, if you experience persistent or severe digestive issues, consult with a healthcare professional.

22. Can I continue with the cleanse if I have dietary restrictions or food allergies?

- The cleanse can be adapted to accommodate dietary restrictions or food allergies by customizing the green smoothie recipes to suit your individual needs. Experiment with alternative ingredients and consult with a healthcare professional if needed.

23. How can I stay motivated and accountable during the cleanse?

- Staying motivated and accountable during the cleanse can be challenging, but setting realistic goals, tracking your progress, and seeking support from friends, family, or online communities can help keep you on track.

24. What should I do if I experience dizziness or lightheadedness during the cleanse?

- If you experience dizziness or lightheadedness, it may be a sign that you need to increase your fluid intake or consume more calories. Be sure to listen to your body and prioritize your health and well-being.

25. Will I experience changes in my skin complexion during the cleanse?

- Many participants report improvements in skin complexion, including clearer skin and a healthy glow, as they progress through the cleanse. Nutrient-rich green smoothies can support skin health from the inside out.

26. Can I consume dairy products while on the cleanse?

   - Dairy products should be avoided during the cleanse, as they can be difficult to digest and may interfere with the detoxification process. Opt for dairy-free alternatives such as almond milk or coconut yogurt instead.

27. How can I prevent feeling bloated or gassy during the cleanse?

   - To prevent bloating or gas, focus on consuming smaller, more frequent meals and snacks throughout the day. Additionally, avoid foods that may exacerbate digestive issues and prioritize hydration to support healthy digestion.

28. Can I do the cleanse if I have a history of eating disorders?

   - Individuals with a history of eating disorders should approach the cleanse with caution and consult with a healthcare professional before starting any new dietary regimen. It's essential to prioritize mental and emotional well-being throughout the cleanse process.

29. What should I do if I experience fatigue or low energy levels during the cleanse?

- If you experience fatigue or low energy levels, prioritize rest, hydration, and nutrient-dense foods to support your body's energy needs. Additionally, consider adjusting your activity level and practicing stress-reducing techniques such as meditation or gentle exercise.

30. Can I consume smoothies made with frozen fruits during the cleanse?

- Yes, you can use frozen fruits in your green smoothies during the cleanse. Frozen fruits are convenient and often more budget-friendly than fresh produce, making them an excellent option for creating delicious and nutritious smoothies.

31. Is it normal to experience changes in mood or emotional fluctuations during the cleanse?

- Yes, it's common to experience changes in mood or emotional fluctuations during the cleanse as the body adjusts to dietary changes and detoxification processes. Practice self-care techniques such as meditation, journaling, or spending time in nature to support emotional well-being.

32. What should I do if I experience persistent or severe symptoms during the cleanse?

- If you experience persistent or severe symptoms such as nausea, vomiting, or diarrhea, discontinue the cleanse and consult with a healthcare professional immediately. Your health and safety are of the utmost importance, so be sure to prioritize your well-being.

33. Can I do the cleanse if I'm on a tight budget?

- Yes, the cleanse can be adapted to accommodate a tight budget by prioritizing affordable ingredients such as seasonal fruits and vegetables, leafy greens, and pantry staples. Additionally, consider purchasing ingredients in bulk or opting for store-brand items to save money.

34. What should I do if I feel overwhelmed or discouraged during the cleanse?

- If you feel overwhelmed or discouraged, reach out to friends, family, or online communities for support and encouragement.

Remember that it's normal to experience ups and downs during the cleanse, and every step forward is a step towards improved health and well-being.

35. Can I continue with the cleanse if I'm traveling or on-the-go?

- Yes, the cleanse can be adapted to accommodate travel or on-the-go lifestyles by prepping green smoothies in advance, packing portable snacks, and prioritizing hydration. With a bit of planning and preparation, you can stay on track with your cleanse goals no matter where life takes you.

36. How can I prevent feeling hungry or deprived during the cleanse?

- To prevent feelings of hunger or deprivation, focus on consuming nutrient-dense foods such as fruits, vegetables, whole grains, and lean proteins. Additionally, incorporate healthy fats and protein-rich snacks into your meals and snacks to keep you feeling satisfied and energized throughout the day.

37. What should I do if I experience cravings for unhealthy foods during the cleanse?

- If you experience cravings for unhealthy foods, try distracting yourself with activities such as walking, reading, or practicing a hobby. Additionally, incorporate healthier alternatives such as fruit-based desserts or raw vegetable snacks to satisfy your cravings in a nutritious way.

38. Can I consume caffeinated beverages such as coffee or tea during the cleanse?

- It's best to avoid caffeinated beverages such as coffee or tea during the cleanse, as they can interfere with the detoxification process and disrupt sleep patterns. Opt for caffeine-free alternatives such as herbal teas or water to stay hydrated and support overall health.

39. What should I do if I experience difficulty sticking to the cleanse guidelines?

- If you experience difficulty sticking to the cleanse guidelines, take a moment to reassess your goals and motivations. Reach out to friends, family, or online communities for support and accountability, and consider adjusting your approach to better suit your individual needs and preferences.

40. How can I transition back to a regular diet after completing the cleanse?

- Transitioning back to a regular diet after completing the cleanse should be done gradually to avoid digestive discomfort or shock to the system. Start by reintroducing whole foods such as fruits, vegetables, lean proteins, and whole grains, and listen to your body's hunger and satiety cues as you adjust to eating a wider variety of foods.

41. Can I repeat the cleanse multiple times for greater benefits?

- While repeating the cleanse multiple times may offer additional benefits, it's essential to listen to your body and prioritize balance and sustainability. Consider incorporating elements of the cleanse into your regular diet and lifestyle to support ongoing health and well-being.

42. What should I do if I have further questions or concerns about the cleanse?

- If you have further questions or concerns about the cleanse, don't hesitate to reach out to a healthcare professional or certified nutritionist for personalized guidance and support. Your health and well-being are my top priorities, and I'm here to help you every step of the way. You can contact me through this email absolutelyglorious79@gmail.com

Chapter 8: Real Stories, Real Results

Inspiring Testimonials from Those Who've Triumphed

In this chapter, I am honored to share inspiring testimonials from individuals who have embarked on the 14-Day Green Smoothie Cleanse and experienced remarkable transformations in their health and well-being. These real stories from real people serve as a testament to the transformative power of nutrition and the resilience of the human spirit.

Testimonial 1: Sarah's Journey to Renewed Energy

Sarah, a busy working mother of two, had struggled with low energy levels and fatigue for years. Despite her best efforts to prioritize her health, the demands of juggling work, family, and household responsibilities left her feeling drained and depleted. Determined to reclaim her vitality, Sarah decided to give the 14-Day Green Smoothie Cleanse a try.

"After just a few days on the cleanse, I noticed a significant difference in my energy levels," Sarah shares. "I no longer felt sluggish and tired all the time; instead, I had a newfound sense of vitality and vigor that I hadn't experienced in years."

As Sarah continued with the cleanse, she found that her energy levels continued to improve, along with other unexpected benefits such as clearer skin and better digestion. "The green smoothies became my go-to source of nourishment, and I found myself craving them more than any unhealthy snacks," she says. "By the end of the 14 days, I felt like a whole new person - energized, radiant, and ready to take on the world!"

Testimonial 2: Mark's Journey to Weight Loss Success

For Mark, struggling with excess weight had been a constant battle that left him feeling frustrated and defeated. Despite trying countless diets and exercise regimens, he found himself unable to shed the pounds and reclaim his health. It wasn't until he discovered the 14-Day Green Smoothie Cleanse that everything changed.

"The cleanse was a game-changer for me," Mark shares. "Not only did I lose weight, but I also felt like I was finally taking control of my health in a way that I never had before."

With each passing day on the cleanse, Mark noticed the number on the scale steadily decreasing, along with inches melting away from his waistline. "The best part was that I never felt deprived or hungry," he says. "The green smoothies kept me satisfied and energized throughout the day, and the pounds just seemed to melt away effortlessly."

By the end of the 14 days, Mark had lost a significant amount of weight and gained a newfound sense of confidence and self-esteem. "The cleanse taught me that I have the power to change my health destiny," he says. "I'm forever grateful for the transformation it's brought into my life."

Testimonial 3: Lisa's Journey to Radiant Health
Lisa had always considered herself to be relatively healthy, but she knew that there was room for improvement in her diet and lifestyle.

Seeking to optimize her health and well-being, she decided to embark on the 14-Day Green Smoothie Cleanse as a way to kickstart her journey to radiant health.

"The cleanse was a revelation for me," Lisa shares. "I had no idea that something as simple as drinking green smoothies could have such a profound impact on my health and vitality."

As Lisa immersed herself in the cleanse, she noticed improvements in her digestion, skin complexion, and overall sense of well-being. "I felt like I was giving my body the nourishment it truly craved," she says. "And the best part was that it was easy and enjoyable to stick with."

By the end of the 14 days, Lisa emerged feeling lighter, brighter, and more vibrant than ever before. "The cleanse was just the beginning of my journey to radiant health," she says. "I now have a newfound appreciation for the power of nutrition to heal and transform lives."

Testimonial 4: James' Quest for Optimal Health
James, a hardworking pizza delivery driver, found himself caught in a cycle of unhealthy

eating habits and sedentary lifestyle. Despite his active job, he struggled with weight gain and low energy levels, often turning to fast food for convenience. Tired of feeling sluggish and overweight, James decided to make a change and embarked on the 14-Day Green Smoothie Cleanse.

"The cleanse was a wake-up call for me," James shares. "I realized that I needed to take control of my health and break free from the cycle of unhealthy eating."

As James committed to drinking green smoothies and making healthier food choices, he noticed a remarkable transformation in his energy levels and overall well-being. "I felt like a new person," he says. "The green smoothies gave me the energy I needed to get through my long shifts, and I no longer felt weighed down by unhealthy food choices."

By the end of the 14 days, James had lost weight, gained muscle tone, and felt more confident and empowered than ever before. "The cleanse taught me that I have the power to change my health destiny," he says. "I'm now committed to making healthier choices for myself and my future."

Testimonial 5: Samantha's Journey to Wellness

Samantha, a dedicated nurse working long hours in a busy hospital, found herself struggling to prioritize her health amidst the demands of her job. Despite her best efforts to eat well and exercise regularly, she often felt exhausted and depleted by the end of her shifts. Determined to take better care of herself, Samantha decided to try the 14-Day Green Smoothie Cleanse.

"The cleanse was a game-changer for me," Samantha shares. "I needed something simple and convenient that would give me the nutrition I needed to thrive in my demanding job."

As Samantha incorporated green smoothies into her daily routine, she noticed a significant improvement in her energy levels, mental clarity, and overall sense of well-being. "I felt like I had a newfound sense of vitality and resilience," she says. "The green smoothies kept me going through long shifts, and I no longer felt drained and exhausted at the end of the day."

By the end of the 14 days, Samantha had experienced a profound transformation in her health and well-being. "The cleanse taught me that self-care is non-negotiable," she says. "I'm now committed to making healthier choices for myself, both on and off the job."

These testimonials are just a glimpse into the transformative power of the 14-Day Green Smoothie Cleanse. From renewed energy and weight loss success to radiant health and vitality, the stories of Sarah, Mark, Lisa, and countless others serve as a testament to the incredible potential that lies within each of us to reclaim our health and well-being.

As you embark on your own journey to wellness, may you draw inspiration from these real stories from these individuals who have triumphed before you. Remember that with dedication, perseverance, and a commitment to self-care, anything is possible.

Chapter 9: 14-Day Cleanse Instructions

Day 1: Detox Kickstart
- Morning Ritual: Start your day with a glass of warm water with lemon to aid digestion and detoxification.
- Breakfast: Begin with a green detox smoothie made with kale, spinach, cucumber, apple, lemon, and ginger.
- Morning Snack: Enjoy a small portion of mixed nuts or a piece of fruit.
- Lunch: Have a light salad with mixed greens, cherry tomatoes, cucumber, bell peppers, and a lean protein source like grilled chicken or tofu.
- Afternoon Snack: Sip on another green detox smoothie or have some raw veggies with hummus.
- Dinner: Prepare a nourishing meal of baked salmon or roasted vegetables with quinoa or brown rice.
- Evening: Wind down with herbal tea or a small bowl of mixed berries for dessert.

Day 2: Cleanse Continues

- Morning Ritual: Start your day with a glass of warm water with lemon to aid digestion and detoxification.
- Breakfast: Opt for a refreshing green smoothie packed with spinach, pineapple, banana, and coconut water.
- Morning Snack: Munch on a small portion of Greek yogurt with a sprinkle of granola.
- Lunch: Enjoy a colorful salad with mixed greens, grated carrots, beetroot, avocado, and grilled shrimp.
- Afternoon Snack: Indulge in a creamy avocado smoothie with almond milk, spinach, banana, and a dash of honey.
- Dinner: Try a hearty vegetable stir-fry with tofu or lean beef, served with brown rice or quinoa.
- Evening: Relax with a cup of chamomile tea or a small piece of dark chocolate.

Day 3: Midweek Refresh

- Morning Ritual: Start your day with a glass of warm water with lemon to aid digestion and detoxification.

- Breakfast: Whip up a vibrant green detox smoothie featuring kale, cucumber, green apple, lime, and mint.
- Morning Snack: Have a handful of almonds or a piece of fruit.
- Lunch: Enjoy a light and flavorful quinoa salad with roasted vegetables and a lemon-tahini dressing.
- Afternoon Snack: Blend up a creamy spinach and mango smoothie with almond milk and a touch of vanilla.
- Dinner: Prepare a grilled chicken breast or baked fish with steamed broccoli and a side of sweet potato.
- Evening: Sip on herbal tea or enjoy a small bowl of sliced melon for dessert.

Day 4-13: Cleanse Continues

- Follow a similar structure to Day 1,2 and 3, incorporating different smoothie recipes, salads, and meals from the Appendix sections.
- Stay hydrated throughout the day by drinking plenty of water, herbal teas, and infused water with fruits or herbs.
- Listen to your body's hunger and fullness cues, eating when you're hungry and stopping when you're satisfied.

- Incorporate gentle physical activity such as walking, yoga, or stretching to support detoxification and overall well-being.
- Get plenty of restorative sleep each night to allow your body to repair and rejuvenate.

Day 14: Reflection and Transition
- Reflect on your experience during the cleanse, noting any changes in energy levels, digestion, mood, or overall well-being.
- Gradually reintroduce foods that were eliminated during the cleanse, paying attention to how your body responds.
- Create a plan for incorporating healthy habits and nourishing foods into your daily routine moving forward.
- Celebrate your commitment to self-care and honor the progress you've made toward supporting your health and wellness goals.

Chapter 10: Wrapping Up Your Journey

Congratulations on completing your 14-day cleanse journey! As you reflect on your accomplishments and consider your next steps, it's essential to recognize the progress you've made and celebrate your dedication to your health and well-being. Here are some reflections and advice to help you wrap up your journey:

1. Celebrate Your Accomplishments: Take a moment to acknowledge and celebrate all that you've achieved during the past 14 days. Whether you've noticed improvements in your energy levels, achieved weight loss goals, or simply developed healthier eating habits, each accomplishment is worth celebrating. Give yourself credit for committing to positive changes and taking steps toward a healthier lifestyle.

2. Reflect on Your Experience: Spend some time reflecting on your experience during the cleanse. Consider how you felt physically,

mentally, and emotionally throughout the process. Take note of any changes you noticed in your body, energy levels, mood, and overall well-being. Reflecting on your experience can help you gain insights into what worked well for you and what areas you may want to focus on moving forward.

3. Set Intentions for the Future: As you transition out of the cleanse, take some time to set intentions for the future. Think about your health and wellness goals and consider how you can continue to support them in the days, weeks, and months ahead. Whether you want to maintain your current habits, build upon them, or make new changes, setting clear intentions can help guide your actions and keep you focused on your goals.

4. Continue Nourishing Your Body: Remember that the journey to health and wellness is ongoing, and it's essential to continue nourishing your body with nutrient-rich foods and hydration. Consider incorporating elements of the cleanse, such as green smoothies and protein-packed meals, into your daily routine to support your overall health and well-being. These foods provide essential

nutrients, promote digestive health, and help maintain energy levels, making them valuable additions to any diet.

5. Listen to Your Body: Pay attention to how your body responds to different foods, activities, and lifestyle choices. Listen to your hunger and fullness cues, honor your cravings in moderation, and prioritize self-care practices that support your physical and emotional well-being. Your body has valuable wisdom to share, so tune in and trust yourself to make choices that honor your health and happiness.

6. Stay Flexible and Adaptive: Remember that health and wellness are not about perfection but about finding balance and consistency in your habits. Stay flexible and adaptive as you navigate your journey, and be willing to adjust your approach as needed. Embrace the journey as a learning experience and be open to exploring new foods, activities, and wellness practices that support your goals.

7. Seek Support and Accountability: Surround yourself with a supportive community of friends, family, or peers who share your health and wellness goals. Seek out accountability

partners, join online forums or support groups, or enlist the help of a health coach or professional to provide guidance and encouragement along the way. Having a support system can make a significant difference in staying motivated and committed to your health journey.

As you wrap up your 14-day cleanse journey, remember that every step you take toward better health and well-being is a step in the right direction. Stay committed to your goals, trust in your ability to create positive change, and continue nurturing yourself with love, kindness, and nourishing foods. Your health and happiness are worth investing in, so keep moving forward with confidence and determination. Best wishes on your continued journey to health and wellness!

Appendix 1: Diverse Green Smoothie Recipes for Your Goals

Anti-Aging Smoothies

1. Avocado Glow Smoothie

Servings: 2
Ingredients:
- 1 ripe avocado
- 2 cups spinach
- 1 cucumber
- 1 banana
- 2 tablespoons chia seeds
- 2 cups almond milk

Instructions:
1. Peel and pit the avocado.
2. Blend all ingredients until smooth.
3. Serve immediately and enjoy.

Nutritional Value per Serving: Calories: 250, Protein: 5g, Fat: 14g, Carbohydrates: 30g, Fiber: 10g

2. Berry Blast Antioxidant Smoothie

Servings: 2

Ingredients:

- 2 cups mixed berries (strawberries, blueberries, raspberries)
- 2 cups spinach
- 1 cup Greek yogurt
- 2 tablespoons honey
- 1 cup almond milk

Instructions:

1. Combine all ingredients in a blender.
2. Blend until smooth and creamy.
3. Pour into glasses and serve.

Nutritional Value per Serving: Calories: 220, Protein: 5g, Fat: 3g, Carbohydrates: 45g, Fiber: 10g

3. Avocado Sunshine Smoothie

Servings: 2

Ingredients:

- 1 ripe avocado
- 2 cups spinach
- 1 cup pineapple chunks
- 1 banana
- Juice of 2 limes
- 2 cups coconut swater

Instructions:

1. Peel and pit the avocado.

2. Blend all ingredients until smooth.

3. Pour into glasses and enjoy.

Nutritional Value per Serving: Calories: 320, Protein: 8g, Fat: 18g, Carbohydrates: 35g, Fiber: 12g

4. Green Goddess Detox Smoothie

Servings: 2

Ingredients:

- 2 cups kale
- 1 cucumber
- 1 green apple
- 1/2 avocado
- Juice of 2 lemons
- 1 cup coconut water

Instructions:

1. Combine all ingredients in a blender.

2. Blend until smooth and creamy.

3. Pour into glasses and serve.

Nutritional Value per Serving: Calories: 250, Protein: 6g, Fat: 5g, Carbohydrates: 40g, Fiber: 8g

5. Avocado Dream Smoothie

Servings: 2

Ingredients:

- 1 ripe avocado
- 2 cups spinach
- 1 cup mango chunks
- 1 cup pineapple chunks
- 2 tablespoons flaxseed
- 2 cups almond milk

Instructions:

1. Peel and pit the avocado.
2. Blend all ingredients until smooth.
3. Divide into glasses and serve.

Nutritional Value per Serving: Calories: 300, Protein: 7g, Fat: 16g, Carbohydrates: 35g, Fiber: 9g

6. Superfood Green Smoothie

Servings: 2

Ingredients:

- 2 cups spinach
- 1 cup kale
- 2 bananas
- 1 avocado
- 4 tablespoons chia seeds
- 2 tablespoons honey
- 2 cups coconut water

Instructions:

1. Combine all ingredients in a blender.
2. Blend until smooth and creamy.

3. Pour into glasses and enjoy.

Nutritional Value per Serving: Calories: 270, Protein: 7g, Fat: 8g, Carbohydrates: 45g, Fiber: 12g

7. Avocado & Almond Delight Smoothie

Servings: 2
Ingredients:
- 1 ripe avocado
- 2 cups spinach
- 1/2 cup almonds
- 1 banana
- 2 tablespoons almond butter
- 2 teaspoons honey
- 2 cups almond milk

Instructions:
1. Peel and pit the avocado.
2. Blend all ingredients until smooth.
3. Divide into glasses and serve.

Nutritional Value per Serving: Calories: 300, Protein: 8g, Fat: 18g, Carbohydrates: 30g, Fiber: 10g

8. Coconut-Kale Green Smoothie

Servings: 2
Ingredients:

- 2 cups kale
- 1 cup coconut milk
- 2 bananas
- 1 cup pineapple chunks
- 2 tablespoons shredded coconut
- Juice of 2 limes

Instructions:

1. Combine all ingredients in a blender.
2. Blend until smooth and creamy.
3. Pour into glasses and enjoy.

Nutritional Value per Serving: Calories: 220, Protein: 5g, Fat: 10g, Carbohydrates: 30g, Fiber: 8g

9. Spinach-Berry Rejuvenation Smoothie

Servings: 2
Ingredients:

- 2 cups spinach
- 1 cup mixed berries (strawberries, blueberries, raspberries)
- 1/2 avocado
- 1 banana
- 1 tablespoon flaxseed
- 1 tablespoon honey
- 1 1/2 cups coconut water

Instructions:

1. Combine all ingredients in a blender.

2. Blend until smooth and creamy.

3. Pour into glasses and enjoy.

Nutritional Value per Serving: Calories: 240, Protein: 5g, Fat: 9g, Carbohydrates: 40g, Fiber: 10g

10. Minty Mango Green Smoothie

Servings: 2

Ingredients:

- 2 cups spinach
- 1 ripe mango, peeled and diced
- 1/2 avocado
- 1/2 cup fresh mint leaves
- Juice of 1 lime
- 1 tablespoon honey
- 1 1/2 cups almond milk

Instructions:

1. Combine all ingredients in a blender.

2. Blend until smooth and creamy.

3. Divide into glasses and serve.

Nutritional Value per Serving: Calories: 280, Protein: 6g, Fat: 11g, Carbohydrates: 45g, Fiber: 10g

11. Kale Cherry Bomb

Servings: 2

Ingredients:

- 1½ cups frozen pitted dark sweet cherries

- 1½ cups unsweetened almond milk
- 1 teaspoon vanilla extract
- 6 kale leaves, washed and de-stemmed
- 1 scoop protein powder (optional)

Instructions:

1. Blend all ingredients until smooth.
2. Pour into glasses and serve.

Nutritional Value per Serving: Calories: 125, Protein: 3g, Carbohydrates: 23g, Fiber: 4g, Sugars: 15g, Fat: 2.5g, Saturated Fat: 0g, Sodium: 148mg

12. Parsley Pizzazz

Servings: 2

Ingredients:

- ½ cup chopped fresh parsley
- 1½ cups frozen mango chunks
- 1 stalk celery
- 2-inch piece of cucumber
- 2 tablespoons fresh lime juice
- 1½ cups coconut water

Instructions:

1. Blend all ingredients until smooth.
2. Pour into glasses and serve.

Nutritional Value per Serving: Calories: 133, Protein: 4g, Carbohydrates: 30g, Fiber: 6g,

Sugars: 22g, Fat: 1g, Saturated Fat: 0.5g, Sodium: 232mg

13. Spring Smoothie

Servings: 2

Ingredients:
- 2 handfuls mixed greens
- Thumb-sized knob fresh ginger
- 1¼ cups frozen peaches
- 1 cup orange juice
- ½ cup water
- 1 cup ice
- 1 teaspoon spirulina (optional)

Instructions:
1. Blend all ingredients until smooth.
2. Pour into glasses and serve.

Nutritional Value per Serving: Calories: 93, Protein: 2g, Carbohydrates: 23g, Fiber: 2g, Sugars: 18g, Fat: 0g, Saturated Fat: 0g, Sodium: 8mg

14. Blueberry Basil Bliss

Servings: 2

Ingredients:
- 5-6 basil leaves
- 1 cup frozen blueberries
- 1¾ cups almond milk

Instructions:

1. Blend all ingredients until smooth.
2. Pour into glasses and serve.

Nutritional Value per Serving: Calories: 70, Protein: 1g, Carbohydrates: 10g, Fiber: 3g, Sugars: 6g, Fat: 3g, Saturated Fat: 0g, Sodium: 158mg

15. Berry Green Blast

Servings: 2

Ingredients:

- 3 large Swiss chard leaves
- 1¼ cups frozen mixed berries
- 1½ cups almond milk
- ½ teaspoon cinnamon
- Handful ice cubes

Instructions:

1. Blend all ingredients until smooth.
2. Pour into glasses and serve.

Nutritional Value per Serving: Calories: 82, Protein: 3g, Carbohydrates: 14g, Fiber: 5g, Sugars: 6g, Fat: 0g, Saturated Fat: 0g, Sodium: 289mg

Bone and Joint Health Smoothies

1. Spinach Strawberry Smoothie

Servings: 2

Ingredients:

- 2 cups fresh spinach
- 1½ cups frozen strawberries
- 1 banana
- 1 cup almond milk
- 1 tablespoon chia seeds

Instructions:

1. Blend all ingredients until smooth.
2. Pour into glasses and serve.

Nutritional Value per Serving: Calories: 135, Protein: 4g, Carbohydrates: 27g, Fiber: 7g, Sugars: 15g, Fat: 4g, Saturated Fat: 0.5g, Sodium: 98mg

2. Kale Pineapple Smoothie

Servings: 2

Ingredients:

- 2 cups chopped kale
- 1½ cups frozen pineapple chunks
- 1 orange, peeled
- 1 tablespoon hemp seeds
- 1 cup coconut water

Instructions:
   1. Blend all ingredients until smooth.
   2. Pour into glasses and serve.

   Nutritional Value per Serving: Calories: 160, Protein: 6g, Carbohydrates: 33g, Fiber: 6g, Sugars: 19g, Fat: 3g, Saturated Fat: 0g, Sodium: 50mg

3. Turmeric Ginger Smoothie
   Servings: 2
   Ingredients:
   - 2 cups spinach
   - 1 banana
   - 1 teaspoon grated fresh turmeric (or ½ teaspoon ground turmeric)
   - 1 teaspoon grated fresh ginger
   - 1 tablespoon flaxseed meal
   - 1 cup unsweetened almond milk
   Instructions:
   1. Blend all ingredients until smooth.
   2. Pour into glasses and serve.

   Nutritional Value per Serving: Calories: 160, Protein: 4g, Carbohydrates: 31g, Fiber: 8g, Sugars: 14g, Fat: 5g, Saturated Fat: 0.5g, Sodium: 100mg

4. Broccoli Berry Blast

Servings: 2

Ingredients:

- 1 cup broccoli florets
- 1 cup mixed berries (strawberries, blueberries, raspberries)
- 1 banana
- 1 tablespoon almond butter
- 1 cup coconut water

Instructions:

1. Blend all ingredients until smooth.
2. Pour into glasses and serve.

Nutritional Value per Serving: Calories: 180, Protein: 5g, Carbohydrates: 35g, Fiber: 8g, Sugars: 20g, Fat: 5g, Saturated Fat: 0.5g, Sodium: 60mg

5. Avocado Almond Smoothie

Servings: 2

Ingredients:

- 1 ripe avocado
- 1 handful spinach
- 1 tablespoon almond butter
- 1 tablespoon honey
- 1½ cups almond milk

Instructions:

1. Blend all ingredients until smooth.

2. Pour into glasses and serve.

Nutritional Value per Serving: Calories: 220, Protein: 5g, Carbohydrates: 18g, Fiber: 9g, Sugars: 6g, Fat: 17g, Saturated Fat: 2g, Sodium: 150mg

6. Collard Green Kiwi Smoothie

Servings: 2
Ingredients:
- 2 collard green leaves
- 2 kiwis, peeled
- 1 banana
- 1 tablespoon chia seeds
- 1 cup coconut water

Instructions:
1. Blend all ingredients until smooth.
2. Pour into glasses and serve.

Nutritional Value per Serving: Calories: 180, Protein: 5g, Carbohydrates: 36g, Fiber: 11g, Sugars: 19g, Fat: 5g, Saturated Fat: 0.5g, Sodium: 50mg

7. Sweet Potato Spice Smoothie

Servings: 2
Ingredients:
- 1 cup cooked sweet potato, cooled

- 1 cup kale
- 1 apple, cored and chopped
- 1 teaspoon ground cinnamon
- 1 tablespoon honey
- 1½ cups almond milk

Instructions:

1. Blend all ingredients until smooth.
2. Pour into glasses and serve.

Nutritional Value per Serving: Calories: 190, Protein: 4g, Carbohydrates: 40g, Fiber: 8g, Sugars: 20g, Fat: 3g, Saturated Fat: 0g, Sodium: 110mg

8. Cherry Almond Greens Smoothie

Servings: 2

Ingredients:

- 1 cup spinach
- 1 cup frozen cherries
- ½ avocado
- 1 tablespoon almond butter
- 1 cup almond milk

Instructions:

1. Blend all ingredients until smooth.
2. Pour into glasses and serve.

Nutritional Value per Serving: Calories: 180, Protein: 5g, Carbohydrates: 23g, Fiber: 8g,

Sugars: 11g, Fat: 9g, Saturated Fat: 1g, Sodium: 120mg

9. Ginger Beet Smoothie

Servings: 2

Ingredients:
- 1 small beet, cooked and peeled
- 1 orange, peeled
- 1-inch piece of fresh ginger
- 1 tablespoon hemp seeds
- 1½ cups coconut water

Instructions:
1. Blend all ingredients until smooth.
2. Pour into glasses and serve.

Nutritional Value per Serving: Calories: 150, Protein: 5g, Carbohydrates: 27g, Fiber: 6g, Sugars: 18g, Fat: 4g, Saturated Fat: 0g, Sodium: 140mg

10. Pineapple Turmeric Green Smoothie

Servings: 2

Ingredients:
- 1 cup kale
- 1 cup pineapple chunks
- ½ teaspoon ground turmeric
- 1 tablespoon flaxseed meal
- 1½ cups coconut water

Instructions:

1. Blend all ingredients until smooth.
2. Pour into glasses and serve.

Nutritional Value per Serving: Calories: 160, Protein: 4g, Carbohydrates: 32g, Fiber: 6g, Sugars: 18g, Fat: 4g, Saturated Fat: 0g, Sodium: 80mg

Constipation Relief Smoothies

1. Prune Power Smoothie
   Servings: 2
   Ingredients:
   - 1 cup pitted prunes
   - 1 ripe banana
   - 1 cup spinach
   - 1 tablespoon flaxseed meal
   - 1½ cups almond milk
   Instructions:
   1. Blend all ingredients until smooth.
   2. Pour into glasses and serve.

Nutritional Value per Serving: Calories: 220, Protein: 5g, Carbohydrates: 40g, Fiber: 10g, Sugars: 20g, Fat: 5g, Saturated Fat: 0.5g, Sodium: 100mg

2. Fiber Booster Smoothie

Servings: 2

Ingredients:
- 1 cup chopped kale
- 1 cup pineapple chunks
- 1 tablespoon chia seeds
- ½ avocado
- 1½ cups coconut water

Instructions:
1. Blend all ingredients until smooth.
2. Pour into glasses and serve.

Nutritional Value per Serving: Calories: 240, Protein: 6g, Carbohydrates: 35g, Fiber: 12g, Sugars: 20g, Fat: 9g, Saturated Fat: 2g, Sodium: 80mg

3. Apple Cinnamon Smoothie

Servings: 2

Ingredients:
- 1 apple, cored and chopped
- 1 tablespoon almond butter
- 1 teaspoon ground cinnamon
- 1 cup spinach
- 1½ cups almond milk

Instructions:
1. Blend all ingredients until smooth.

2. Pour into glasses and serve.

Nutritional Value per Serving: Calories: 180, Protein: 4g, Carbohydrates: 30g, Fiber: 8g, Sugars: 18g, Fat: 7g, Saturated Fat: 1g, Sodium: 120mg

4. Papaya Passion Smoothie

Servings: 2

Ingredients:
- 1 cup chopped papaya
- 1 ripe banana
- 1 cup kale
- 1 tablespoon honey
- 1½ cups coconut water

Instructions:
1. Blend all ingredients until smooth.
2. Pour into glasses and serve.

Nutritional Value per Serving: Calories: 210, Protein: 3g, Carbohydrates: 45g, Fiber: 10g, Sugars: 30g, Fat: 2g, Saturated Fat: 1g, Sodium: 60mg

5. Berry Blast Smoothie

Servings: 2

Ingredients:

- 1 cup mixed berries (strawberries, blueberries, raspberries)
- 1 ripe banana
- 1 tablespoon flaxseed meal
- 1 cup spinach
- 1½ cups almond milk

Instructions:

1. Blend all ingredients until smooth.
2. Pour into glasses and serve.

Nutritional Value per Serving: Calories: 200, Protein: 5g, Carbohydrates: 35g, Fiber: 10g, Sugars: 20g, Fat: 6g, Saturated Fat: 0.5g, Sodium: 100mg

6. Kiwi Kale Smoothie

Servings: 2

Ingredients:

- 2 kiwis, peeled
- 1 cup chopped kale
- 1 ripe avocado
- 1 tablespoon chia seeds
- 1½ cups coconut water

Instructions:

1. Blend all ingredients until smooth.
2. Pour into glasses and serve.

Nutritional Value per Serving: Calories: 250, Protein: 5g, Carbohydrates: 35g, Fiber: 12g, Sugars: 18g, Fat: 10g, Saturated Fat: 1.5g, Sodium: 70mg

7. Mango Mint Smoothie

Servings: 2

Ingredients:
- 1 cup frozen mango chunks
- 1 handful fresh mint leaves
- 1 banana
- 1 tablespoon hemp seeds
- 1½ cups almond milk

Instructions:
1. Blend all ingredients until smooth.
2. Pour into glasses and serve.

Nutritional Value per Serving: Calories: 230, Protein: 5g, Carbohydrates: 35g, Fiber: 8g, Sugars: 20g, Fat: 7g, Saturated Fat: 0.5g, Sodium: 100mg

8. Fig and Flax Smoothie

Servings: 2

Ingredients:
- 1 cup dried figs, soaked in water overnight
- 1 ripe banana
- 1 cup spinach

- 1 tablespoon ground flaxseed
- 1½ cups almond milk

Instructions:
1. Blend all ingredients until smooth.
2. Pour into glasses and serve.

Nutritional Value per Serving: Calories: 220, Protein: 4g, Carbohydrates: 40g, Fiber: 10g, Sugars: 25g, Fat: 6g, Saturated Fat: 0.5g, Sodium: 120mg

9. Pear Power Smoothie

Servings: 2

Ingredients:
- 1 ripe pear, cored and chopped
- 1 cup Swiss chard leaves
- 1 tablespoon almond butter
- 1 teaspoon grated ginger
- 1½ cups coconut water

Instructions:
1. Blend all ingredients until smooth.
2. Pour into glasses and serve.

Nutritional Value per Serving: Calories: 230, Protein: 4g, Carbohydrates: 40g, Fiber: 9g, Sugars: 25g, Fat: 8g, Saturated Fat: 1g, Sodium: 90mg

10. Carrot Cake Smoothie

Servings: 2

Ingredients:

- 1 cup grated carrots
- 1 ripe banana
- 1 tablespoon almond butter
- ½ teaspoon ground cinnamon
- 1 cup spinach
- 1½ cups almond milk

Instructions:

1. Blend all ingredients until smooth.
2. Pour into glasses and serve.

Nutritional Value per Serving: Calories: 210, Protein: 5g, Carbohydrates: 35g, Fiber: 9g, Sugars: 18g, Fat: 7g, Saturated Fat: 0.5g, Sodium: 110mg

Stress-Busting Smoothies

1. Calm and Cool Smoothie

Servings: 2

Ingredients:

- 1 cup spinach
- 1 frozen banana
- 1/2 cup sliced cucumber
- 1 tablespoon fresh mint leaves

- 1 tablespoon honey
- 1 cup coconut water

Instructions:

1. Blend all ingredients until smooth.

2. Pour into glasses and garnish with mint leaves if desired.

Nutritional Value per Serving: Calories: 95, Protein: 2g, Carbohydrates: 24g, Fiber: 3g, Sugars: 16g, Fat: 0g, Sodium: 80mg

2. Tranquil Tropical Smoothie

Servings: 2

Ingredients:

- 1 cup kale
- 1/2 cup frozen pineapple chunks
- 1/2 cup frozen mango chunks
- 1 tablespoon coconut flakes
- 1 tablespoon chia seeds
- 1 cup coconut water

Instructions:

1. Blend all ingredients until smooth.

2. Pour into glasses and sprinkle with additional coconut flakes on top.

Nutritional Value per Serving: Calories: 150, Protein: 4g, Carbohydrates: 25g, Fiber: 7g, Sugars: 16g, Fat: 5g, Sodium: 15mg

3. Serenity Spinach Smoothie

Servings: 2

Ingredients:

- 2 cups spinach
- 1/2 ripe avocado
- 1/2 cup frozen berries (such as blueberries or raspberries)
- 1 tablespoon almond butter
- 1 tablespoon honey
- 1 cup almond milk

Instructions:

1. Blend all ingredients until smooth.
2. Pour into glasses and enjoy.

Nutritional Value per Serving: Calories: 220, Protein: 5g, Carbohydrates: 20g, Fiber: 7g, Sugars: 11g, Fat: 15g, Sodium: 120mg

4. Peaceful Pear Smoothie

Servings: 2

Ingredients:

- 1 cup Swiss chard leaves
- 1 ripe pear, cored and chopped
- 1/2 ripe banana
- 1 tablespoon fresh ginger, grated
- 1 tablespoon lemon juice
- 1 cup water

Instructions:
1. Blend all ingredients until smooth.
2. Pour into glasses and garnish with a slice of pear if desired.

Nutritional Value per Serving: Calories: 120, Protein: 2g, Carbohydrates: 30g, Fiber: 5g, Sugars: 17g, Fat: 0g, Sodium: 20mg

5. Zen Zucchini Smoothie

Servings: 2

Ingredients:
- 1 cup zucchini, chopped
- 1/2 cup frozen green grapes
- 1/2 cup fresh spinach
- 1 tablespoon fresh basil leaves
- 1 tablespoon honey
- 1 cup coconut water

Instructions:
1. Blend all ingredients until smooth.
2. Pour into glasses and enjoy the refreshing taste.

Nutritional Value per Serving: Calories: 90, Protein: 2g, Carbohydrates: 20g, Fiber: 3g, Sugars: 15g, Fat: 0g, Sodium: 50mg

6. Relaxation Raspberry Smoothie

Servings: 2

Ingredients:

- 1 cup spinach
- 1/2 cup frozen raspberries
- 1/2 ripe avocado
- 1 tablespoon hemp seeds
- 1 tablespoon honey
- 1 cup almond milk

Instructions:

1. Blend all ingredients until smooth.

2. Pour into glasses and savor the berry goodness.

Nutritional Value per Serving: Calories: 210, Protein: 6g, Carbohydrates: 25g, Fiber: 8g, Sugars: 15g, Fat: 11g, Sodium: 110mg

7. Blissful Blueberry Smoothie

Servings: 2

Ingredients:

- 1 cup kale
- 1/2 cup frozen blueberries
- 1/2 cup cucumber, sliced
- 1 tablespoon fresh mint leaves
- 1 tablespoon honey
- 1 cup coconut water

Instructions:

1. Blend all ingredients until smooth.

2. Pour into glasses and enjoy the calming effects of blueberries and mint.

Nutritional Value per Serving: Calories: 100, Protein: 3g, Carbohydrates: 20g, Fiber: 4g, Sugars: 13g, Fat: 0g, Sodium: 80mg

8. Mellow Mango Smoothie

Servings: 2

Ingredients:
- 1 cup spinach
- 1/2 cup frozen mango chunks
- 1/2 ripe banana
- 1 tablespoon almond butter
- 1 tablespoon honey
- 1 cup almond milk

Instructions:
1. Blend all ingredients until smooth.

2. Pour into glasses and relax with this tropical delight.

Nutritional Value per Serving: Calories: 220, Protein: 6g, Carbohydrates: 30g, Fiber: 6g, Sugars: 20g, Fat: 8g, Sodium: 120mg

9. Stress-Free Strawberry Smoothie

Servings: 2

Ingredients:
- 1 cup Swiss chard leaves
- 1/2 cup frozen strawberries
- 1/2 ripe avocado
- 1 tablespoon chia seeds
- 1 tablespoon honey
- 1 cup coconut water

Instructions:

1. Blend all ingredients until smooth.

2. Pour into glasses and unwind with this nutritious treat.

Nutritional Value per Serving: Calories: 180, Protein: 5g, Carbohydrates: 25g, Fiber: 7g, Sugars: 14g, Fat: 9g, Sodium: 110mg

10. Tranquility Turmeric Smoothie

Servings: 2

Ingredients:
- 1 cup kale
- 1/2 cup frozen pineapple chunks
- 1/2 inch fresh turmeric root, peeled
- 1 tablespoon coconut flakes
- 1 tablespoon honey
- 1 cup coconut water

Instructions:

1. Blend all ingredients until smooth.

2. Pour into glasses and enjoy the calming benefits of turmeric.

Nutritional Value per Serving: Calories: 120, Protein: 3g, Carbohydrates: 25g, Fiber: 5g, Sugars: 15g, Fat: 3g, Sodium: 60mg

Immune Boosting Smoothies

1. Immune Booster Green Smoothie
   Servings: 2
   Ingredients:
   - 2 cups spinach
   - 1 ripe banana
   - 1 cup pineapple chunks
   - 1-inch piece of ginger, peeled
   - 1 tablespoon honey (optional)
   - 1 cup coconut water
   Instructions:
   1. Combine all ingredients in a blender.
   2. Blend until smooth and creamy.
   3. Taste and adjust sweetness with honey, if desired.
   4. Pour into glasses and serve.

Nutritional Value (per serving): 150 cal, 3g protein, 35g carbohydrates, 5g fiber, 25g sugars, 1g fat, 0g saturated fat, 50mg sodium

2. Tropical Tiger Nut Smoothie

Servings: 2

Ingredients:

- 1 ripe mango, peeled and diced
- 1/2 cup pineapple chunks
- 2 tablespoons tiger nut flour or soaked tiger nuts
- 1/2 cup coconut water
- 1/2 cup Greek yogurt
- Handful of spinach or kale

Instructions:

1. Place all ingredients in a blender.
2. Blend until smooth and creamy.
3. Adjust consistency by adding more coconut water if needed.
4. Pour into glasses and enjoy!

3. Antioxidant Green Smoothie

Servings: 2

Ingredients:

- 2 cups spinach
- 1 cup mixed berries (such as strawberries, blueberries, raspberries)
- 1/2 avocado

- 1 tablespoon hemp seeds
- 1 tablespoon honey (optional)
- 1 cup almond milk (or any milk of choice)

Instructions:

1. Combine all ingredients in a blender.
2. Blend until smooth and creamy.
3. Adjust sweetness with honey, if desired.
4. Pour into glasses and serve.

Nutritional Value (per serving): 180 cal, 5g protein, 25g carbohydrates, 8g fiber, 15g sugars, 7g fat, 1g saturated fat, 70mg sodium

4. Tropical Green Immune Boost Smoothie

Servings: 2

Ingredients:

- 2 cups spinach
- 1/2 cup frozen mango chunks
- 1/2 cup frozen pineapple chunks
- 1 kiwi, peeled
- 1 tablespoon fresh lime juice
- 1 cup coconut water

Instructions:

1. Place all ingredients in a blender.
2. Blend until smooth and creamy.
3. Adjust consistency by adding more coconut water if needed.
4. Pour into glasses and enjoy.

Nutritional Value (per serving): 140 cal, 3g protein, 30g carbohydrates, 6g fiber, 20g sugars, 1g fat, 0g saturated fat, 45mg sodium

5. Super Green Immunity Booster

Servings: 2

Ingredients:

- 2 cups kale
- 1 green apple, cored and chopped
- 1/2 cucumber, chopped
- 1 tablespoon fresh lemon juice
- 1 tablespoon fresh ginger, grated
- 1 cup water or coconut water

Instructions:

1. Combine all ingredients in a blender.
2. Blend until smooth and creamy.
3. Adjust flavor with more lemon juice or ginger, if desired.
4. Pour into glasses and serve.

Nutritional Value (per serving): 120 kcal, 3g protein, 25g carbohydrates, 5g fiber, 15g sugars, 1g fat, 0g saturated fat, 30mg sodium

6. Berry Kale Immunity Booster

Servings: 2

Ingredients:

- 2 cups kale
- 1/2 cup mixed berries (strawberries, blueberries, raspberries)
- 1/2 cup Greek yogurt (or dairy-free yogurt)
- 1 tablespoon honey (optional)
- 1 tablespoon chia seeds
- 1 cup almond milk (or any milk of choice)

Instructions:

1. Place all ingredients in a blender.
2. Blend until smooth and creamy.
3. Adjust sweetness with honey, if desired.
4. Pour into glasses and enjoy.

Nutritional Value (per serving): 170 cal, 7g protein, 30g carbohydrates, 8g fiber, 15g sugars, 3g fat, 0.5g saturated fat, 60mg sodium

7. Ginger Turmeric Immune Boost Smoothie

Servings: 2

Ingredients:

- 2 cups spinach
- 1 banana
- 1/2 teaspoon grated ginger
- 1/2 teaspoon ground turmeric
- 1 tablespoon honey (optional)
- 1 cup coconut water or water

Instructions:

1. Combine all ingredients in a blender.

2. Blend until smooth and creamy.

3. Adjust sweetness with honey, if desired.

4. Pour into glasses and serve.

Nutritional Value (per serving): 160 cal, 3g protein, 35g carbohydrates, 6g fiber, 20g sugars, 1g fat, 0g saturated fat, 50mg sodium

8. Avocado Green Immunity Smoothie

Servings: 2

Ingredients:

- 1 ripe avocado
- 2 cups spinach
- 1 green apple, cored and chopped
- 1/2 cup cucumber, chopped
- 1 tablespoon fresh lemon juice
- 1 cup coconut water or water

Instructions:

1. Place all ingredients in a blender.

2. Blend until smooth and creamy.

3. Adjust flavor with more lemon juice, if desired.

4. Pour into glasses and enjoy.

Nutritional Value (per serving): 180 cal, 3g protein, 20g carbohydrates, 8g fiber, 10g sugars, 9g fat, 1g saturated fat, 40mg sodium

9. Matcha Green Tea Immune Booster

Servings: 2

Ingredients:
- 2 cups spinach
- 1 teaspoon matcha green tea powder
- 1/2 cup frozen mango chunks
- 1/2 cup pineapple chunks
- 1 tablespoon honey (optional)
- 1 cup almond milk (or any milk of choice)

Instructions:
1. Combine all ingredients in a blender.
2. Blend until smooth and creamy.
3. Adjust sweetness with honey, if desired.
4. Pour into glasses and serve.

Nutritional Value (per serving): 150 cal, 3g protein, 30g carbohydrates, 5g fiber, 20g sugars, 2g fat, 0g saturated fat, 60mg sodium

10. Spirulina Superfood Smoothie

Servings: 2

Ingredients:
- 2 cups kale
- 1 banana
- 1 tablespoon spirulina powder
- 1/2 cup frozen pineapple chunks
- 1 tablespoon honey (optional)
- 1 cup coconut water or water

Instructions:
1. Place all ingredients in a blender.
2. Blend until smooth and creamy.
3. Adjust sweetness with honey, if desired.
4. Pour into glasses and enjoy.

Nutritional Value (per serving): 160 cal, 3g protein, 35g carbohydrates, 6g fiber, 20g sugars, 1.5g fat, 0.5g saturated fat, 50mg sodium

11. Tiger Nut Berry Blast Smoothie

Servings: 2

Ingredients:
- 1 cup mixed berries (such as strawberries, blueberries, raspberries)
- 1 ripe banana
- 2 tablespoons tiger nut flour or soaked tiger nuts
- 1 cup spinach
- 1 cup almond milk (or tiger nut milk for extra flavor)
- Ice cubes (optional)

Instructions:
1. Combine all ingredients in a blender.
2. Blend until smooth and creamy.
3. Add ice cubes if desired for a colder texture.

4. Pour into glasses and serve immediately.

Nutritional Value (per serving): 140 cal, 3g protein, 28g carbohydrates, 6g fiber, 15g sugars, 3g fat, 0.5g saturated fat, 80mg sodium

12. Citrus Green Immunity Smoothie

Servings: 2

Ingredients:

- 2 cups kale
- 1 orange, peeled and segmented
- 1/2 cup pineapple chunks
- 1/2 cup Greek yogurt (or dairy-free yogurt)
- 1 tablespoon chia seeds
- 1 cup water or coconut water

Instructions:

1. Place all ingredients in a blender.
2. Blend until smooth and creamy.
3. Add more water if needed to reach desired consistency.
4. Pour into glasses and enjoy.

Nutritional Value (per serving): 160 cal, 6g protein, 30g carbohydrates, 8g fiber, 15g sugars, 3g fat, 0.5g saturated fat, 60mg sodium

Heart Health Smoothies

1. Heart Healthy Green Smoothie

Servings: 2

Ingredients:
- 2 cups kale
- 1 ripe banana
- 1/2 cup strawberries
- 1 tablespoon flax seeds
- 1 tablespoon honey (optional)
- 1 cup almond milk (or any milk of choice)

Instructions:
1. Combine all ingredients in a blender.
2. Blend until smooth and creamy.
3. Adjust sweetness with honey, if desired.
4. Pour into glasses and serve.

Nutritional Value (per serving): 150 cal, 4g protein, 25g carbohydrates, 6g fiber, 15g sugars, 5g fat, 0.5g saturated fat, 70mg sodium

2. Avocado Berry Heart Smoothie

Servings: 2

Ingredients:
- 1/2 ripe avocado
- 1 cup spinach

- 1/2 cup mixed berries (raspberries, blueberries)
- 1 tablespoon chia seeds
- 1 tablespoon honey (optional)
- 1 cup coconut water or water

Instructions:

1. Place all ingredients in a blender.
2. Blend until smooth and creamy.
3. Adjust sweetness with honey, if desired.
4. Pour into glasses and enjoy.

Nutritional Value (per serving): 170 cal, 4g protein, 20g carbohydrates, 8g fiber, 10g sugars, 9g fat, 1g saturated fat, 40mg sodium

3. Green Tea Heart Smoothie

Servings: 2

Ingredients:

- 2 cups spinach
- 1 ripe pear, cored and chopped
- 1 tablespoon green tea powder (matcha)
- 1 tablespoon honey (optional)
- 1/2 cup Greek yogurt (or dairy-free yogurt)
- 1 cup almond milk (or any milk of choice)

Instructions:

1. Combine all ingredients in a blender.
2. Blend until smooth and creamy.
3. Adjust sweetness with honey, if desired.

4. Pour into glasses and serve.

Nutritional Value (per serving): 160 cal, 6g protein, 30g carbohydrates, 6g fiber, 15g sugars, 3g fat, 0.5g saturated fat, 70mg sodium

4. Beetroot Kale Heart Smoothie

Servings: 2

Ingredients:
- 2 cups kale
- 1 small cooked beetroot, chopped
- 1/2 cup pineapple chunks
- 1 tablespoon hemp seeds
- 1 tablespoon honey (optional)
- 1 cup coconut water or water

Instructions:
1. Place all ingredients in a blender.
2. Blend until smooth and creamy.
3. Adjust sweetness with honey, if desired.
4. Pour into glasses and enjoy.

Nutritional Value (per serving): 150 cal, 5g protein, 30g carbohydrates, 7g fiber, 15g sugars, 4g fat, 0.5g saturated fat, 60mg sodium

5. Spinach Blueberry Heart Smoothie

Servings: 2

Ingredients:

- 2 cups spinach
- 1/2 cup blueberries (fresh or frozen)
- 1/2 ripe banana
- 1 tablespoon flaxseeds
- 1 tablespoon honey (optional)
- 1 cup almond milk (or any milk of choice)

Instructions:

1. Combine all ingredients in a blender.
2. Blend until smooth and creamy.
3. Adjust sweetness with honey, if desired.
4. Pour into glasses and serve.

Nutritional Value (per serving): 140 cal, 3g protein, 25g carbohydrates, 6g fiber, 15g sugars, 4.5g fat, 0.5g saturated fat, 70mg sodium

6. Green Berry Cardio Smoothie

Servings: 2

Ingredients:

- 2 cups baby spinach
- 1/2 cup mixed berries (strawberries, blueberries, raspberries)
- 1/2 ripe banana
- 1 tablespoon flax seeds
- 1 tablespoon honey (optional)
- 1 cup unsweetened almond milk (or any milk of choice)

Instructions:
1. Combine all ingredients in a blender.
2. Blend until smooth and creamy.
3. Adjust sweetness with honey, if desired.
4. Pour into glasses and serve.

Nutritional Value (per serving): 130 cal, 3g protein, 25g carbohydrates, 6g fiber, 15g sugars, 3.5g fat, 0.5g saturated fat, 70mg sodium

7. Kiwi Spinach Heart Smoothie
Servings: 2
Ingredients:
- 2 cups spinach
- 2 ripe kiwis, peeled and sliced
- 1/2 ripe avocado
- 1 tablespoon honey (optional)
- Juice of 1 lime
- 1 cup coconut water or water

Instructions:
1. Combine all ingredients in a blender.
2. Blend until smooth and creamy.
3. Adjust sweetness with honey, if desired.
4. Pour into glasses and enjoy.

Nutritional Value (per serving): 170 cal, 3g protein, 25g carbohydrates, 7g fiber, 15g sugars, 6g fat, 1g saturated fat, 70mg sodium

8. Pomegranate Green Heart Smoothie

Servings: 2

Ingredients:
- 2 cups baby spinach
- 1/2 cup pomegranate seeds
- 1/2 cup cucumber, chopped
- 1/2 cup Greek yogurt (or dairy-free yogurt)
- 1 tablespoon honey (optional)
- 1 cup almond milk (or any milk of choice)

Instructions:
1. Place all ingredients in a blender.
2. Blend until smooth and creamy.
3. Adjust sweetness with honey, if desired.
4. Pour into glasses and serve.

Nutritional Value (per serving): 140 cal, 5g protein, 20g carbohydrates, 5g fiber, 12g sugars, 4.5g fat, 0.5g saturated fat, 70mg sodium

9. Minty Beet Heart Smoothie

Servings: 2

Ingredients:
- 1 cup beet greens

- 1 small cooked beetroot, chopped
- Handful of fresh mint leaves
- 1/2 cup frozen raspberries
- 1 tablespoon honey (optional)
- 1 cup coconut water or water
- Instructions:
    1. Combine all ingredients in a blender.
    2. Blend until smooth and creamy.
    3. Adjust sweetness with honey, if desired.
    4. Pour into glasses and enjoy.

Nutritional Value (per serving): 160 cal, 4g protein, 30g carbohydrates, 7g fiber, 15g sugars, 5g fat, 0.5g saturated fat, 60mg sodium

10. Spinach Mango Heart Smoothie

Servings: 2

Ingredients:
- 2 cups spinach
- 1 ripe mango, peeled and chopped
- 1/2 cup pineapple chunks
- 1 tablespoon chia seeds
- 1 tablespoon honey (optional)
- 1 cup almond milk (or any milk of choice)

Instructions:
    1. Place all ingredients in a blender.
    2. Blend until smooth and creamy.
    3. Adjust sweetness with honey, if desired.

4. Pour into glasses and serve.

Nutritional Value (per serving): 150 cal, 3g protein, 25g carbohydrates, 6g fiber, 15g sugars, 4.5g fat, 0.5g saturated fat, 70mg sodium

Detoxification Smoothies

1. Green Goddess Detox Smoothie
Servings: 2
Ingredients:
- 2 cups spinach
- 1/2 cucumber, chopped
- 1/2 avocado
- 1/2 lemon, juiced
- 1 tablespoon fresh ginger, grated
- 1 cup coconut water

Instructions:
1. Combine all ingredients in a blender.
2. Blend until smooth and creamy.
3. Pour into glasses and serve.

Nutritional Value (per serving): 140 cal, 3g protein, 12g carbohydrates, 7g fiber, 3g sugars, 9g fat, 1g saturated fat, 90mg sodium

2. Cleansing Green Apple Smoothie

Servings: 2

Ingredients:

- 2 cups kale
- 1 green apple, cored and chopped
- 1/2 cucumber, chopped
- 1/2 lemon, juiced
- 1 tablespoon fresh parsley
- 1 cup coconut water

Instructions:

1. Place all ingredients in a blender.
2. Blend until smooth and creamy.
3. Pour into glasses and serve.

Nutritional Value (per serving): 120 cal, 2.5g protein, 14g carbohydrates, 5g fiber, 7g sugars, 7g fat, 1g saturated fat, 80mg sodium

3. Detoxifying Green Pineapple Smoothie

Servings: 2

Ingredients:

- 2 cups spinach
- 1 cup pineapple chunks
- 1/2 banana
- 1/2 inch fresh ginger, grated
- 1 tablespoon chia seeds
- 1 cup coconut water

Instructions:

1. Combine all ingredients in a blender.
2. Blend until smooth and creamy.
3. Pour into glasses and serve.

Nutritional Value (per serving): 150 cal, 3g protein, 25g carbohydrates, 6g fiber, 15g sugars, 4g fat, 0.5g saturated fat, 70mg sodium

4. Refreshing Green Detox Smoothie

Servings: 2
Ingredients:
- 2 cups Swiss chard
- 1/2 cucumber, chopped
- 1/2 cup fresh mint leaves
- 1/2 lime, juiced
- 1/2 cup coconut water
- 1/2 cup ice cubes

Instructions:
1. Place all ingredients in a blender.
2. Blend until smooth and creamy.
3. Pour into glasses and serve.

Nutritional Value (per serving): 80 cal, 2g protein, 16g carbohydrates, 5g fiber, 6g sugars, 1.5g fat, 0.5g saturated fat, 40mg sodium

5. Detox Green Grape Smoothie

Servings: 2

Ingredients:
  - 2 cups spinach
  - 1 cup green grapes
  - 1/2 avocado
  - 1/2 lemon, juiced
  - 1 tablespoon fresh cilantro
  - 1 cup coconut water

Instructions:
  1. Combine all ingredients in a blender.
  2. Blend until smooth and creamy.
  3. Pour into glasses and serve.

Nutritional Value (per serving): 140 cal, 2.5g protein, 16g carbohydrates, 5g fiber, 9g sugars, 8g fat, 1g saturated fat, 70mg sodium

6. Alkalizing Green Detox Smoothie

Servings: 2

Ingredients:
  - 2 cups kale
  - 1/2 cup cucumber, chopped
  - 1/2 green apple, cored and chopped
  - 1/2 lemon, juiced
  - 1 tablespoon fresh parsley
  - 1 cup coconut water

Instructions:
  1. Place all ingredients in a blender.
  2. Blend until smooth and creamy.

3. Pour into glasses and serve.

Nutritional Value (per serving): 130 cal, 2.5g protein, 14g carbohydrates, 5g fiber, 7g sugars, 7g fat, 1g saturated fat, 80mg sodium

7. Detox Green Tea Smoothie

Servings: 2

Ingredients:
- 2 cups baby spinach
- 1/2 cup brewed green tea, chilled
- 1/2 cup pineapple chunks
- 1/2 banana
- 1 tablespoon fresh mint leaves
- 1/2 tablespoon honey (optional)

Instructions:
1. Combine all ingredients in a blender.
2. Blend until smooth and creamy.
3. Pour into glasses and serve.

Nutritional Value (per serving): 120 cal, 2.5g protein, 26g carbohydrates, 4g fiber, 17g sugars, 1g fat, 0.5g saturated fat, 60mg sodium

8. Detoxifying Green Mango Smoothie

Servings: 2

Ingredients:
- 2 cups spinach

- 1 cup chopped mango
- 1/2 cucumber, chopped
- 1/2 lime, juiced
- 1 tablespoon fresh cilantro
- 1 cup coconut water

Instructions:

1. Combine all ingredients in a blender.
2. Blend until smooth and creamy.
3. Pour into glasses and serve.

Nutritional Value (per serving): 140 cal, 3g protein, 28g carbohydrates, 6g fiber, 18g sugars, 4g fat, 0.5g saturated fat, 70mg sodium

9. Ginger Detox Green Smoothie

Servings: 2

Ingredients:

- 2 cups kale
- 1/2 cup chopped pineapple
- 1/2 banana
- 1/2 inch fresh ginger, grated
- 1 tablespoon chia seeds
- 1 cup coconut water

Instructions:

1. Combine all ingredients in a blender.
2. Blend until smooth and creamy.
3. Pour into glasses and serve.

Nutritional Value (per serving): 150 cal, 3g protein, 28g carbohydrates, 7g fiber, 15g sugars, 5g fat, 1g saturated fat, 80mg sodium

10. Detoxifying Green Lemonade Smoothie
Servings: 2
Ingredients:
- 2 cups spinach
- 1/2 cucumber, chopped
- 1/2 lemon, juiced
- 1/2 green apple, cored and chopped
- 1 tablespoon fresh parsley
- 1 cup coconut water

Instructions:
1. Combine all ingredients in a blender.
2. Blend until smooth and creamy.
3. Pour into glasses and serve.

Nutritional Value (per serving): 130 cal, 3g protein, 16g carbohydrates, 6g fiber, 8g sugars, 5g fat, 1g saturated fat, 70mg sodium

Energy-Boosting Smoothies

1. Orange Spinach Banana Smoothie
Servings: 2
Ingredients:

- 2 cups spinach
- 1 orange, peeled and segmented
- 1 banana
- 1/2 cup Greek yogurt
- 1 tablespoon honey
- 1/2 cup almond milk

Instructions:

1. Combine all ingredients in a blender.
2. Blend until smooth and creamy.
3. Pour into glasses and serve.

Nutritional Value (per serving): 160 cal, 5g protein, 35g carbohydrates, 6g fiber, 24g sugars, 1.5g fat, 0.5g saturated fat, 80mg sodium

2. Banana Cucumber Mango Green Smoothie

Servings: 2

Ingredients:

- 2 cups spinach
- 1/2 cucumber, chopped
- 1 ripe banana
- 1 cup chopped mango
- 1 tablespoon chia seeds
- 1 cup coconut water

Instructions:

1. Place all ingredients in a blender.
2. Blend until smooth and creamy.

3. Pour into glasses and serve.

Nutritional Value (per serving): 170 cal, 4g protein, 32g carbohydrates, 7g fiber, 20g sugars, 5g fat, 0.5g saturated fat, 70mg sodium

3. Vanilla Green Tea Smoothie

Servings: 2

Ingredients:
- 2 cups spinach
- 1 cup brewed green tea, chilled
- 1/2 cup plain Greek yogurt
- 1/2 teaspoon vanilla extract
- 1 tablespoon honey
- 1 banana

Instructions:
1. Combine all ingredients in a blender.
2. Blend until smooth and creamy.
3. Pour into glasses and serve.

Nutritional Value (per serving): 150 cal, 6g protein, 30g carbohydrates, 5g fiber, 20g sugars, 1.5g fat, 0.5g saturated fat, 70mg sodium

4. Berry Blast Energy Smoothie

Servings: 2

Ingredients:

- 1 cup spinach
- 1/2 cup strawberries
- 1/2 cup blueberries
- 1/2 cup raspberries
- 1 banana
- 1 tablespoon honey
- 1 cup almond milk

Instructions:

1. Place all ingredients in a blender.
2. Blend until smooth and creamy.
3. Pour into glasses and serve.

Nutritional Value (per serving): 180 cal, 4g protein, 40g carbohydrates, 8g fiber, 25g sugars, 2.5g fat, 0.5g saturated fat, 90mg sodium

5. Pineapple Coconut Green Smoothie:

Servings: 2

Ingredients:

- 2 cups spinach
- 1 cup chopped pineapple
- 1/2 banana
- 1/4 cup coconut flakes
- 1 tablespoon honey
- 1 cup coconut water

Instructions:

1. Combine all ingredients in a blender.
2. Blend until smooth and creamy.
3. Pour into glasses and serve.

Nutritional Value (per serving): 190 cal, 3g protein, 35g carbohydrates, 6g fiber, 25g sugars, 3.5g fat, 2.5g saturated fat, 100mg sodium

6. Minty Green Citrus Smoothie

Servings: 2
Ingredients:
- 2 cups spinach
- 1 orange, peeled and segmented
- 1/2 banana
- 1/4 cup fresh mint leaves
- 1 tablespoon honey
- 1 cup orange juice

Instructions:
1. Place all ingredients in a blender.
2. Blend until smooth and creamy.
3. Pour into glasses and serve.

Nutritional Value (per serving): 170 cal, 3g protein, 38g carbohydrates, 6g fiber, 25g sugars, 1.5g fat, 0.5g saturated fat, 10mg sodium

7. Avocado Green Power Smoothie

Servings: 2

Ingredients:

- 2 cups spinach
- 1/2 ripe avocado
- 1 banana
- 1 tablespoon almond butter
- 1 tablespoon honey
- 1 cup almond milk

Instructions:

1. Combine all ingredients in a blender.
2. Blend until smooth and creamy.
3. Pour into glasses and serve.

Nutritional Value (per serving): 200 cal, 5g protein, 25g carbohydrates, 8g fiber, 15g sugars, 8g fat, 1g saturated fat, 80mg sodium

8. Matcha Green Energy Smoothie

Servings: 2

Ingredients:

- 2 cups spinach
- 1 teaspoon matcha powder
- 1/2 cup Greek yogurt
- 1 tablespoon honey
- 1 cup coconut water

Instructions:

1. Place all ingredients in a blender.

2. Blend until smooth and creamy.
3. Pour into glasses and serve.

Nutritional Value (per serving): 170 cal, 6g protein, 35g carbohydrates, 5g fiber, 25g sugars, 1.5g fat, 0.5g saturated fat, 70mg sodium

9. Kiwi Green Energy Smoothie
Servings: 2
Ingredients:
  - 2 cups spinach
  - 2 kiwis, peeled and sliced
  - 1/2 banana
  - 1/2 cup pineapple chunks
  - 1 tablespoon honey
  - 1 cup coconut water

Instructions:
  1. Combine all ingredients in a blender.
  2. Blend until smooth and creamy.
  3. Pour into glasses and serve.

Nutritional Value (per serving): 180 cal, 3g protein, 40g carbohydrates, 7g fiber, 25g sugars, 2g fat, 0.5g saturated fat, 60mg sodium

10. Green Protein Power Smoothie
Servings: 2

Ingredients:

- 2 cups spinach
- 1 scoop vanilla protein powder
- 1 banana
- 1 tablespoon almond butter
- 1 tablespoon honey
- 1 cup almond milk

Instructions:

1. Combine all ingredients in a blender.
2. Blend until smooth and creamy.
3. Pour into glasses and serve.

Nutritional Value (per serving): 220 cal, 12g protein, 30g carbohydrates, 6g fiber, 20g sugars, 6g fat, 1g saturated fat, 90mg sodium

11. Pomegranate Green Smoothie

Servings: 2

Ingredients:

- 2 cups spinach
- 1/2 cup pomegranate seeds
- 1 banana
- 1/2 cup Greek yogurt
- 1 tablespoon honey
- 1 cup coconut water

Instructions:

1. Place all ingredients in a blender.
2. Blend until smooth and creamy.

3. Pour into glasses and serve.

Nutritional Value (per serving): 190 cal, 5g protein, 40g carbohydrates, 7g fiber, 30g sugars, 1.5g fat, 0.5g saturated fat, 70mg sodium

12. Matcha Pear Green Smoothie

Servings: 2

Ingredients:
- 2 cups spinach
- 1 ripe pear, cored and chopped
- 1 teaspoon matcha green tea powder
- 1 banana
- 1 tablespoon honey
- 1 cup almond milk

Instructions:
1. Combine all ingredients in a blender.
2. Blend until smooth and creamy.
3. Pour into glasses and serve.

Nutritional Value (per serving): 190 cal, 4g protein, 40g carbohydrates, 6g fiber, 26g sugars, 2g fat, 0.5g saturated fat, 80mg sodium

Beauty Enhancing Smoothies

1. Tropical Paradise Smoothie

Servings: 2

Ingredients:

- 1 cup spinach
- 1 tablespoon flax seeds, grounded
- 1/2 cup pineapple chunks
- 1/2 cup mango chunks
- 1 handful of almonds
- ½ cup papaya
- 1/2 cup coconut water
- Juice of 1 lime

Instructions:

1. Combine all ingredients in a blender.
2. Blend until smooth and creamy.
3. Pour into glasses and serve.

Nutritional Value (per serving): 150 cal, 2g protein, 35g carbohydrates, 5g fiber, 25g sugars, 1g fat, 0g saturated fat, 60mg sodium

2. Orange Creamsicle Smoothie Recipe

Servings: 2

Ingredients:

- 2 cups spinach
- 1 orange, peeled and segmented
- 1/2 cup Greek yogurt
- 1 medium sized carrot
- 1/2 teaspoon vanilla extract

- 1 tablespoon honey
- 1 tablespoon turmeric powder
- 1/2 cup unsweetened coconut milk

Instructions:
1. Combine all ingredients in a blender.
2. Blend until smooth and creamy.
3. Pour into glasses and serve.

Nutritional Value (per serving): 160 cal, 6g protein, 30g carbohydrates, 4g fiber, 22g sugars, 2g fat, 0.5g saturated fat, 70mg sodium

3. Chocolate Lovers Smoothie

Servings: 2

Ingredients:
- 2 cups spinach
- 2 tablespoons unsweetened cocoa powder
- 1/2 avocado
- 1 handful of walnuts
- 1 tablespoon honey
- ½ cup strawberries
- 1 cup almond milk
- 1 tablespoon chia seeds

Instructions:
1. Combine all ingredients in a blender.
2. Blend until smooth and creamy.
3. Pour into glasses and serve.

Nutritional Value (per serving): 180 cal, 4g protein, 35g carbohydrates, 7g fiber, 20g sugars, 3.5g fat, 1g saturated fat, 60mg sodium

4. Berry Beauty Blast

Servings: 2
Ingredients:
- 1 cup spinach
- 1/2 cup strawberries
- 1/2 cup blueberries
- 1/2 cup raspberries
- 1 banana
- 1/2 cup Greek yogurt
- 1 tablespoon honey
- 1/2 cup coconut water

Instructions:
1. Combine all ingredients in a blender.
2. Blend until smooth and creamy.
3. Pour into glasses and serve.

Nutritional Value (per serving): 170 cal, 5g protein, 35g carbohydrates, 7g fiber, 25g sugars, 1g fat, 0.5g saturated fat, 50mg sodium

5. Green Goddess Glow

Servings: 2
Ingredients:

- 2 cups spinach
- 1/2 cucumber, peeled and sliced
- 1 kiwi, peeled and sliced
- 1/2 avocado
- Juice of 1 lime
- 1 tablespoon honey
- 1/2 cup coconut water

Instructions:

1. Combine all ingredients in a blender.
2. Blend until smooth and creamy.
3. Pour into glasses and serve.

Nutritional Value (per serving): 160 cal, 3g protein, 30g carbohydrates, 7g fiber, 20g sugars, 3.5g fat, 0.5g saturated fat, 60mg sodium

6. Radiant Raspberry Refresher

Servings: 2

Ingredients:

- 1 cup spinach
- 1/2 cup raspberries
- 1/2 cup strawberries
- 1 banana
- 1/2 cup Greek yogurt
- 1 tablespoon honey
- 1/2 cup almond milk

Instructions:

1. Combine all ingredients in a blender.
2. Blend until smooth and creamy.
3. Pour into glasses and serve.

Nutritional Value (per serving): 150 cal, 4g protein, 30g carbohydrates, 6g fiber, 22g sugars, 1.5g fat, 0.5g saturated fat, 60mg sodium

7. Golden Glow Smoothie

Servings: 2
Ingredients:
- 2 cups spinach
- 1/2 cup pineapple chunks
- 1/2 cup mango chunks
- 1 banana
- 1/2 teaspoon turmeric
- 1/2 cup coconut water

Instructions:
1. Combine all ingredients in a blender.
2. Blend until smooth and creamy.
3. Pour into glasses and serve.

Nutritional Value (per serving): 160 cal, 2g protein, 35g carbohydrates, 5g fiber, 25g sugars, 1g fat, 0g saturated fat, 60mg sodium

8. Citrus Sunshine Smoothie

Servings: 2
Ingredients:
- 2 cups spinach
- 1 orange, peeled and segmented
- 1/2 cup pineapple chunks
- 1 banana
- Juice of 1 lime
- 1 tablespoon honey
- 1/2 cup coconut water

Instructions:
1. Combine all ingredients in a blender.
2. Blend until smooth and creamy.
3. Pour into glasses and serve.

Nutritional Value (per serving): 150 cal, 2g protein, 35g carbohydrates, 5g fiber, 25g sugars, 1g fat, 0g saturated fat, 60mg sodium

9. Berry Avocado Boost

Servings: 2
Ingredients:
- 1 cup spinach
- 1/2 avocado
- 1/2 cup strawberries
- 1/2 cup blueberries
- 1 banana
- 1 tablespoon honey
- 1/2 cup almond milk

Instructions:
1. Combine all ingredients in a blender.
2. Blend until smooth and creamy.
3. Pour into glasses and serve.

Nutritional Value (per serving): 180 cal, 3g protein, 35g carbohydrates, 7g fiber, 20g sugars, 4g fat, 1g saturated fat, 60mg sodium

10. Coconut Kale Dream

Servings: 2

Ingredients:
- 2 cups kale
- 1/2 cup coconut milk
- 1/2 cup pineapple chunks
- 1 banana
- 1/2 teaspoon vanilla extract
- 1 tablespoon honey

Instructions:
1. Combine all ingredients in a blender.
2. Blend until smooth and creamy.
3. Pour into glasses and serve.

Nutritional Value (per serving): 170 cal, 3g protein, 35g carbohydrates, 5g fiber, 25g sugars, 3.5g fat, 1g saturated fat, 60mg sodium

Blood Sugar Control Smoothies

1. Green Apple Cinnamon Delight
Servings: 2
Ingredients:
- 2 cups spinach
- 1 green apple, chopped
- 1/2 teaspoon cinnamon
- 1/2 avocado
- 1 tablespoon chia seeds
- 1 cup unsweetened almond milk

Instructions:
1. Combine all ingredients in a blender.
2. Blend until smooth and creamy.
3. Pour into glasses and serve.

Nutritional Value (per serving): 170 cal, 3g protein, 25g carbohydrates, 9g fiber, 12g sugars, 8g fat, 1g saturated fat, 80mg sodium

2. Spinach Berry Blast
Servings: 2
Ingredients:
- 2 cups spinach
- 1/2 cup strawberries
- 1/2 cup blueberries
- 1/2 cup raspberries

- 1/2 banana
- 1 tablespoon flaxseed meal
- 1 cup unsweetened coconut water

Instructions:

1. Combine all ingredients in a blender.
2. Blend until smooth and creamy.
3. Pour into glasses and serve.

Nutritional Value (per serving): 150 cal, 3g protein, 30g carbohydrates, 8g fiber, 15g sugars, 4.5g fat, 0.5g saturated fat, 70mg sodium

3. Avocado Spinach Power Smoothie

Servings: 2

Ingredients:

- 2 cups spinach
- 1/2 avocado
- 1/2 cucumber, peeled and sliced
- 1/2 cup Greek yogurt
- 1 tablespoon almond butter
- 1 teaspoon honey
- Juice of 1/2 lemon
- 1 cup unsweetened almond milk

Instructions:

1. Combine all ingredients in a blender.
2. Blend until smooth and creamy.
3. Pour into glasses and serve.

Nutritional Value (per serving): 190 cal, 6g protein, 15g carbohydrates, 6g fiber, 6g sugars, 10g fat, 1g saturated fat, 100mg sodium

4. Kale Berry Smoothie

Servings: 2

Ingredients:

- 2 cups kale
- 1/2 cup strawberries
- 1/2 cup raspberries
- 1/2 cup blueberries
- 1/2 banana
- 1 tablespoon hemp seeds
- 1 cup unsweetened coconut water

Instructions:

1. Combine all ingredients in a blender.
2. Blend until smooth and creamy.
3. Pour into glasses and serve.

Nutritional Value (per serving): 140 cal, 4g protein, 25g carbohydrates, 8g fiber, 12g sugars, 5g fat, 0.5g saturated fat, 60mg sodium

5. Ginger Green Smoothie

Servings: 2

Ingredients:

- 2 cups spinach

- 1/2 avocado
- 1/2 inch fresh ginger, peeled
- 1/2 cup cucumber, peeled and sliced
- 1/2 cup pineapple chunks
- 1 tablespoon chia seeds
- 1 cup unsweetened almond milk

Instructions:

1. Combine all ingredients in a blender.
2. Blend until smooth and creamy.
3. Pour into glasses and serve.

Nutritional Value (per serving): 180 cal, 4g protein, 20g carbohydrates, 9g fiber, 10g sugars, 9g fat, 1g saturated fat, 70mg sodium

6. Berry Spinach Protein Smoothie

Servings: 2

Ingredients:

- 2 cups spinach
- 1/2 cup mixed berries (strawberries, blueberries, raspberries)
- 1/2 banana
- 1/2 cup Greek yogurt
- 1 tablespoon almond butter
- 1 scoop protein powder (vanilla or unflavored)
- 1 cup unsweetened almond milk

Instructions:

1. Combine all ingredients in a blender.
2. Blend until smooth and creamy.
3. Pour into glasses and serve.

Nutritional Value (per serving): 200 cal, 12g protein, 20g carbohydrates, 6g fiber, 10g sugars, 8g fat, 1g saturated fat, 90mg sodium

7. Turmeric Mango Smoothie

Servings: 2

Ingredients:
- 2 cups spinach
- 1/2 cup frozen mango chunks
- 1/2 banana
- 1/2 teaspoon ground turmeric
- 1 tablespoon flaxseed meal
- 1 cup unsweetened coconut water

Instructions:
1. Combine all ingredients in a blender.
2. Blend until smooth and creamy.
3. Pour into glasses and serve.

Nutritional Value (per serving): 160 cal, 3g protein, 25g carbohydrates, 8g fiber, 15g sugars, 6g fat, 0.5g saturated fat, 80mg sodium

8. Green Tea Berry Smoothie

Servings: 2

Ingredients:
- 2 cups baby spinach
- 1/2 cup mixed berries (strawberries, raspberries, blackberries)
- 1/2 banana
- 1/2 cup brewed green tea, cooled
- 1 tablespoon honey
- 1/2 cup unsweetened almond milk

Instructions:
1. Combine all ingredients in a blender.
2. Blend until smooth and creamy.
3. Pour into glasses and serve.

Nutritional Value (per serving): 140 cal, 2g protein, 30g carbohydrates, 7g fiber, 18g sugars, 3g fat, 0.5g saturated fat, 70mg sodium

9. Avocado Berry Smoothie

Servings: 2

Ingredients:
- 2 cups spinach
- 1/2 avocado
- 1/2 cup mixed berries (blueberries, raspberries)
- 1/2 banana
- 1 tablespoon hemp seeds
- 1 cup unsweetened coconut water

Instructions:

1. Combine all ingredients in a blender.
2. Blend until smooth and creamy.
3. Pour into glasses and serve.

Nutritional Value (per serving): 170 cal, 4g protein, 20g carbohydrates, 7g fiber, 10g sugars, 9g fat, 1g saturated fat, 60mg sodium

10. Pineapple Ginger Green Smoothie

Servings: 2

Ingredients:
- 2 cups kale
- 1/2 cup pineapple chunks
- 1/2 inch fresh ginger, peeled
- 1/2 cucumber, peeled and sliced
- 1/2 cup coconut water
- Juice of 1/2 lime

Instructions:
1. Combine all ingredients in a blender.
2. Blend until smooth and creamy.
3. Pour into glasses and serve.

Nutritional Value (per serving): 150 cal, 3g protein, 30g carbohydrates, 8g fiber, 15g sugars, 5g fat, 0.5g saturated fat, 60mg sodium

Fat Burning Smoothies

1. Purple Passion Green Smoothie

Ingredients:
- ½ cup strawberries
- ¼ cup blueberries
- 1 cup raw spinach
- ¼ cup Greek yogurt
- 1 cup water

Instructions:
1. Add all ingredients to a blender.
2. Blend until smooth, adding more water as needed.
3. Serve immediately.

Nutritional Value (per serving): Calories: 286, Fat: 0.5g, Saturated Fat: 0g, Fiber: 3g, Protein: 44g, Carbohydrates: 28.3g

2. Grown-Up Strawberry Banana Green Smoothie

Ingredients:
- ½ cup strawberries
- 1 banana
- 1 cup raw spinach
- ½ cup almond milk
- 1 teaspoon vanilla extract

Instructions:
   1. Add all ingredients to a blender.
   2. Blend until smooth, adjusting thickness with water if necessary.
   3. Serve immediately.

   Nutritional Value (per serving): Calories: 207, Fat: 3.2g, Saturated Fat: 0g, Fiber: 5.2g, Protein: 3.6g, Carbohydrates: 42.1g

3. Apple Pie Green Smoothie
Ingredients:
   - 1 apple, peeled and cored
   - ¼ cup blueberries
   - ¼ teaspoon cinnamon
   - ⅛ teaspoon nutmeg
   - 1 cup spinach
   - 1 tablespoon chia seeds
   - 1 teaspoon vanilla extract
   - 1 cup water
  - Instructions:
   1. Combine all ingredients in a blender.
   2. Blend until smooth and creamy.
   3. Serve immediately.

   Nutritional Value (per serving): Calories: 165, Fat: 5.3g, Saturated Fat: 0.4g, Fiber: 11.4g, Protein: 4.1g, Carbohydrates: 34g

4. Electric Green Boost

Ingredients:
- ¼ cup pineapple
- 1 orange, peeled
- 1 cup raw spinach
- 1 cup almond milk

Instructions:
1. Combine all ingredients in a blender.
2. Blend until smooth and creamy.
3. Serve immediately.

Nutritional Value (per serving): Calories: 174, Fat: 2.9g, Saturated Fat: 0.1g, Fiber: 5.7g, Protein: 3.8g, Carbohydrates: 36.1g

5. Sweetie Pea Green Smoothie

Ingredients:
- 1 cup sweet peas
- 1 banana
- ½ cup blueberries
- 1 cup almond milk
- 1 tablespoon chia seeds
- ½ teaspoon honey

Instructions:
1. Combine all ingredients in a blender.
2. Blend until smooth and creamy.
3. Serve immediately.

Nutritional Value (per serving): Calories: 393, Fat: 8.7g, Saturated Fat: 0.6g, Fiber: 17.2g, Protein: 13.7g, Carbohydrates: 75.3g

6. Crisp Mango Cucumber Green Smoothie

Ingredients:
- ¼ cup mango
- 1 orange, peeled
- 1 cup chopped cucumber
- 1 tablespoon flax seeds
- 1 cup spinach

Instructions:
1. Combine all ingredients in a blender.
2. Blend until smooth and creamy.
3. Serve immediately.

Nutritional Value (per serving): Calories: 153, Fat: 2.8g, Saturated Fat: 0.4g, Fiber: 6.8g, Protein: 4.5g, Carbohydrates: 30.7g

7. Green Tropical Sunrise

Ingredients:
- ¼ cup pineapple
- 1 orange, peeled
- 1 carrot
- 1 cup spinach
- 1 tablespoon flax seeds

- 1 cup water

Instructions:

1. Combine all ingredients in a blender.
2. Blend until smooth and creamy.
3. Serve immediately.

Nutritional Value (per serving): Calories: 176, Fat: 2.6g, Saturated Fat: 0.4g, Fiber: 9.1g, Protein: 4.6g, Carbohydrates: 36.1g

8. Citrus Spinach Detox Smoothie

Ingredients:

- 1 orange, peeled and segmented
- ½ grapefruit, peeled and segmented
- 1 cup spinach
- ½ cucumber, peeled and chopped
- 1 tablespoon fresh mint leaves
- 1 tablespoon chia seeds
- 1 cup coconut water

Instructions:

1. Combine all ingredients in a blender.
2. Blend until smooth and creamy.
3. Serve immediately.

Nutritional Value (per serving): Calories: 215, Fat: 4.6g, Saturated Fat: 0.6g, Fiber: 10.2g, Protein: 6.1g, Carbohydrates: 41.5g

9. Pineapple Ginger Green Smoothie
Ingredients:
- 1 cup pineapple chunks
- 1-inch piece of fresh ginger, peeled
- 1 cup spinach
- Juice of ½ lime
- 1 tablespoon chia seeds
- 1 cup coconut water

Instructions:
1. Combine all ingredients in a blender.
2. Blend until smooth and creamy.
3. Serve immediately.

Nutritional Value (per serving): Calories: 186, Fat: 3.8g, Saturated Fat: 0.4g, Fiber: 8.9g, Protein: 5.1g, Carbohydrates: 35.4g

10. Avocado Kale Detox Smoothie
Ingredients:
- ½ avocado
- 1 cup kale
- ½ cucumber
- 1 tablespoon fresh mint leaves
- Juice of 1 lemon
- 1 tablespoon hemp seeds
- 1 cup coconut water

Instructions:
1. Combine all ingredients in a blender.

2. Blend until smooth and creamy.

3. Serve immediately.

Nutritional Value (per serving): Calories: 225, Fat: 13.4g, Saturated Fat: 1.8g, Fiber: 9.5g, Protein: 7.2g, Carbohydrates: 23.6g

11. Spinach Pineapple Protein Smoothie

Ingredients:
- 1 cup spinach
- 1 cup pineapple chunks
- ½ cup plain Greek yogurt
- 1 scoop vanilla protein powder
- 1 tablespoon flax seeds
- 1 cup unsweetened almond milk

Instructions:
1. Combine all ingredients in a blender.
2. Blend until smooth and creamy.
3. Serve immediately.

Nutritional Value (per serving): Calories: 308, Fat: 6.9g, Saturated Fat: 0.7g, Fiber: 7.8g, Protein: 33.6g, Carbohydrates: 33.7g

12. Mango Spinach Green Smoothie

Ingredients:
- 1 cup spinach
- 1 cup mango chunks

- ½ banana
- 1 tablespoon almond butter
- 1 tablespoon chia seeds
- 1 cup coconut water

Instructions:
1. Combine all ingredients in a blender.
2. Blend until smooth and creamy.
3. Serve immediately.

Nutritional Value (per serving): Calories: 286, Fat: 8.7g, Saturated Fat: 0.7g, Fiber: 9.8g, Protein: 8.5g, Carbohydrates: 48.2g

Miscellaneous Health Boosting Smoothies

1. Turmeric Ginger Immunity Booster
Ingredients:
- 1 banana
- 1 cup pineapple chunks
- 1 teaspoon turmeric powder
- ½ teaspoon grated ginger
- 1 tablespoon honey
- 1 cup coconut water

Instructions:
1. Combine all ingredients in a blender.

2. Blend until smooth and creamy.

3. Serve chilled.

Nutritional Value (per serving): Calories: 195, Fat: 0.6g, Saturated Fat: 0g, Fiber: 4.2g, Protein: 1.5g, Carbohydrates: 50.3g

2. Beetroot Berry Bliss

Ingredients:

- 1 small beetroot, cooked and chopped
- 1 cup mixed berries (strawberries, raspberries, blueberries)
- ½ cup Greek yogurt
- 1 tablespoon honey
- 1 cup almond milk

Instructions:

1. Combine all ingredients in a blender.

2. Blend until smooth and creamy.

3. Garnish with fresh berries before serving.

Nutritional Value (per serving): Calories: 198, Fat: 2.4g, Saturated Fat: 0.3g, Fiber: 5.9g, Protein: 9.8g, Carbohydrates: 33.7g

3. Minty Melon Refresher

Ingredients:

- 2 cups chopped honeydew melon
- ½ cup cucumber, peeled and chopped

- ¼ cup fresh mint leaves
- Juice of 1 lime
- 1 tablespoon agave nectar
- 1 cup coconut water

Instructions:

1. Combine all ingredients in a blender.
2. Blend until smooth and creamy.
3. Serve over ice cubes.

Nutritional Value (per serving): Calories: 123, Fat: 0.5g, Saturated Fat: 0g, Fiber: 2.5g, Protein: 1.5g, Carbohydrates: 31.7g

4. Chia Seed Berry Blast

Ingredients:

- 1 cup mixed berries (strawberries, blueberries, raspberries)
- 1 tablespoon chia seeds
- ½ cup Greek yogurt
- 1 tablespoon honey
- 1 cup almond milk

Instructions:

1. Combine all ingredients in a blender.
2. Blend until smooth and creamy.
3. Let sit for 5 minutes to allow chia seeds to expand before serving.

Nutritional Value (per serving): Calories: 182, Fat: 2.6g, Saturated Fat: 0.3g, Fiber: 8.9g, Protein: 10.2g, Carbohydrates: 30.4g

5. Avocado Spinach Power Smoothie

Ingredients:
- 1 ripe avocado, peeled and pitted
- 2 cups fresh spinach leaves
- 1 banana
- Juice of 1 lemon
- 1 tablespoon honey
- 1 cup coconut water

Instructions:
1. Combine all ingredients in a blender.
2. Blend until smooth and creamy.
3. Serve immediately.

Nutritional Value (per serving): Calories: 272, Fat: 15.4g, Saturated Fat: 2.3g, Fiber: 9.6g, Protein: 5.1g, Carbohydrates: 34.6g

6. Pineapple Kale Energizer

Ingredients:
- 1 cup pineapple chunks
- 1 cup chopped kale leaves
- ½ banana
- 1 tablespoon flax seeds
- 1 tablespoon honey

- 1 cup coconut water

Instructions:

1. Combine all ingredients in a blender.
2. Blend until smooth and creamy.
3. Serve chilled.

Nutritional Value (per serving): Calories: 204, Fat: 2.8g, Saturated Fat: 0.3g, Fiber: 6.2g, Protein: 4.6g, Carbohydrates: 42.1g

7. Coconut Mango Delight

Ingredients:

- 1 ripe mango, peeled and pitted
- ½ cup coconut milk
- ½ cup Greek yogurt
- 1 tablespoon shredded coconut
- 1 tablespoon honey
- Juice of 1 lime

Instructions:

1. Combine all ingredients in a blender.
2. Blend until smooth and creamy.
3. Garnish with a sprinkle of shredded coconut before serving.

Nutritional Value (per serving): Calories: 292, Fat: 10.4g, Saturated Fat: 8.6g, Fiber: 3.2g, Protein: 10.1g, Carbohydrates: 44.8g

8. Kiwi Basil Zinger

Ingredients:

- 2 kiwi fruits, peeled and chopped
- ½ cup fresh basil leaves
- ½ cup cucumber, peeled and chopped
- Juice of 1 lemon
- 1 tablespoon honey
- 1 cup coconut water

Instructions:

1. Combine all ingredients in a blender.
2. Blend until smooth and creamy.
3. Serve over ice cubes.

Nutritional Value (per serving): Calories: 138, Fat: 0.7g, Saturated Fat: 0.1g, Fiber: 5.1g, Protein: 2.5g, Carbohydrates: 32.4g

Appendix 2: Clean Protein-Packed Meals to Fuel Your Body

Welcome to Appendix B, where you will be provided with a collection of delicious and nutrient-dense recipes to support your journey of fueling your body with clean, protein-packed meals. Whether you're looking to build muscle, support your active lifestyle, or simply maintain a balanced diet, these recipes are designed to provide you with the protein and nutrients your body needs to thrive.

1. Quinoa Power Bowl (Serving Size: 1 bowl)
Ingredients:
- 1 cup cooked quinoa
- 1 cup mixed greens
- ½ cup chickpeas, drained and rinsed
- ¼ cup diced cucumber
- ¼ cup diced tomato
- ¼ cup shredded carrots
- 2 tablespoons pumpkin seeds
- 2 tablespoons crumbled feta cheese
- 2 tablespoons balsamic vinaigrette

Instructions:
1. In a bowl, put the cooked quinoa and mixed greens in layers.
2. Top with chickpeas, cucumber, tomato, shredded carrots, pumpkin seeds, and crumbled feta cheese.
3. Drizzle with balsamic vinaigrette before serving.

Nutritional Value (per serving): Calories: 380, Protein: 16g, Fat: 12g, Carbohydrates: 55g, Fiber: 9g

2. Grilled Lemon Herb Chicken (Serving Size: 1 chicken breast)
Ingredients:
- 4 boneless, skinless chicken breasts
- 2 tablespoons olive oil
- Juice of 1 lemon
- 2 cloves garlic, minced
- 1 teaspoon dried oregano
- 1 teaspoon dried thyme
- Salt and pepper to taste

Instructions:
1. In a bowl, whisk olive oil, lemon juice, minced garlic, dried oregano, dried thyme, salt, and pepper.

2. Place chicken breasts in a shallow dish and pour the marinade over them. Cover and refrigerate for at least 30 minutes.

3. Preheat the grill to medium-high heat. Remove chicken from marinade and discard any excess marinade.

4. Grill chicken for 6-8 minutes per side, or until cooked through and no longer pink in the center.

5. Remove from the grill and let rest for a few minutes before serving.

Nutritional Value (per serving): Calories: 240, Protein: 30g, Fat: 10g, Carbohydrates: 2g, Fiber: 0g

3. Quinoa Stuffed Bell Peppers (Serving Size: 1 stuffed pepper)

Ingredients:
- 4 large bell peppers, any color
- 1 cup cooked quinoa
- 1 cup black beans, drained and rinsed
- 1 cup diced tomatoes
- ½ cup diced onion
- ½ cup corn kernels
- 1 teaspoon chili powder
- ½ teaspoon cumin
- Salt and pepper to taste

- ½ cup shredded cheddar cheese
- Fresh cilantro, for garnish

Instructions:
1. Preheat your oven to 375°F (190°C). Slice the tops off the bell peppers and remove the seeds and membranes.
2. In a big bowl, combine cooked quinoa, black beans, diced tomatoes, onion, corn kernels, chili powder, cumin, salt, and pepper.
3. Stuff each bell pepper with the quinoa mixture and place inside a baking dish.
4. Sprinkle shredded cheddar cheese on top of each stuffed pepper.
5. Cover the baking dish with aluminum foil and bake for 25-30 minutes, or until peppers are tender.
6. Remove foil and bake for an additional 5 minutes to melt the cheese.
7. Garnish with fresh cilantro before serving.

Nutritional Value (per serving): Calories: 290, Protein: 12g, Fat: 6g, Carbohydrates: 50g, Fiber: 10g

4. Greek Yogurt Parfait (Serving Size: 1 parfait)
Ingredients:

- 1 cup Greek yogurt
- ½ cup mixed berries (strawberries, blueberries, raspberries)
- ¼ cup granola
- 1 tablespoon honey
- Fresh mint leaves, for garnish

Instructions:
1. In a glass or bowl, layer Greek yogurt, mixed berries, and granola.
2. Drizzle honey over the top of the parfait.
3. Garnish with fresh mint leaves before serving.

Nutritional Value (per serving): Calories: 280, Protein: 18g, Fat: 6g, Carbohydrates: 40g, Fiber: 6g

5. Salmon Avocado Salad (Serving Size: 1 salad)
Ingredients:
- 4 oz grilled or baked salmon fillet
- 2 cups mixed greens
- ½ avocado, sliced
- ½ cup cherry tomatoes, halved
- ¼ cup sliced cucumber
- 2 tablespoons sliced red onion
- 1 tablespoon olive oil

- 1 tablespoon balsamic vinegar
- Salt and pepper

Instructions:
1. In a big bowl, add the mixed greens, sliced avocado, cherry tomatoes, sliced cucumber, and sliced red onion.
2. Top with grilled or baked salmon fillet.
3. Drizzle olive oil and balsamic vinegar over the salad.
4. Season with salt and pepper before serving.

Nutritional Value (per serving): Calories: 350, Protein: 25g, Fat: 22g, Carbohydrates: 14g, Fiber: 7g

6. Turkey and Vegetable Stir-Fry (Serving Size: 1 plate)
Ingredients:
- 4 oz turkey breast, sliced
- 1 cup mixed vegetables (bell peppers, broccoli, carrots, snap peas)
- 2 cloves garlic, minced
- 1 tablespoon olive oil
- 2 tablespoons low-sodium soy sauce
- 1 teaspoon sesame oil
- 1 teaspoon cornstarch
- Cooked brown rice or quinoa, for serving

Instructions:

1. In a small bowl, whisk together soy sauce, sesame oil, and cornstarch to make the sauce. Set aside.

2. Heat olive oil in a large skillet or wok over medium-high heat. Add minced garlic and cook for 1 minute until fragrant.

3. Add sliced turkey breast to the skillet and cook until browned, about 3-4 minutes.

4. Add mixed vegetables to the skillet and stir-fry for another 3-4 minutes, until vegetables are tender-crisp.

5. Pour the prepared sauce over the turkey and vegetables. Stir well to coat everything evenly and cook for another 2 minutes.

6. Serve the turkey and vegetable stir-fry over cooked brown rice or quinoa.

Nutritional Value (per serving): Calories: 320, Protein: 25g, Fat: 12g, Carbohydrates: 28g, Fiber: 5g

7. Lentil and Vegetable Soup (Serving Size: 1 bowl)

Ingredients:

- 1 cup cooked lentils
- 2 cups vegetable broth

- 1 cup diced tomatoes
- 1 cup diced carrots
- 1 cup diced celery
- 1 cup chopped spinach
- 1 onion, diced
- 2 cloves garlic, minced
- 1 teaspoon olive oil
- 1 teaspoon dried thyme
- Salt and pepper to taste

Instructions:

1. Heat olive oil in a large pot over medium heat. Add diced onion and minced garlic, and cook until softened, about 3-4 minutes.

2. Add diced carrots and celery to the pot, and cook for another 5 minutes.

3. Pour in vegetable broth and diced tomatoes. Bring the mixture to a boil, then reduce heat to low and simmer for 15 minutes.

4. Add cooked lentils and chopped spinach to the pot. Stir well and cook for an additional 5 minutes until heated through.

5. Season the lentil and vegetable soup with dried thyme, salt, and pepper before serving.

Nutritional Value (per serving): Calories: 280, Protein: 18g, Fat: 3g, Carbohydrates: 50g, Fiber: 18g

8. Tofu and Vegetable Skewers (Serving Size: 1 skewer)

Ingredients:
- 4 oz extra-firm tofu, cut into cubes
- 1 cup mixed vegetables (bell peppers, zucchini, cherry tomatoes, mushrooms)
- 2 tablespoons soy sauce
- 1 tablespoon olive oil
- 1 tablespoon maple syrup or honey
- 1 clove garlic, minced
- 1 teaspoon grated ginger
- Wooden skewers, soaked in water for 30 minutes

Instructions:
1. In a small bowl, whisk together soy sauce, olive oil, maple syrup (or honey), minced garlic, and grated ginger to make the marinade.
2. Thread cubes of tofu and mixed vegetables onto the soaked wooden skewers.
3. Place the skewers in a shallow dish and pour the marinade over them, making sure everything is coated evenly. Marinate for at least 30 minutes.
4. Preheat the grill or grill pan to medium-high heat. Grill the skewers for 3-4 minutes on each

side, observing carefully until the vegetables are tender and tofu is lightly charred.

5. Serve the tofu and vegetable skewers hot off the grill.

Nutritional Value (per serving): Calories: 220, Protein: 14g, Fat: 10g, Carbohydrates: 20g, Fiber: 4g

9. Chickpea and Spinach Curry (Serving Size: 1 bowl)

Ingredients:
- 1 can (15 oz) chickpeas, drained and rinsed
- 2 cups chopped spinach
- 1 onion, diced
- 2 cloves garlic, minced
- 1 tablespoon olive oil
- 1 can (14 oz) diced tomatoes
- 1 can (14 oz) coconut milk
- 2 teaspoons curry powder
- 1 teaspoon ground turmeric
- Salt and pepper to taste
- Cooked brown rice, for serving

Instructions:
1. Heat olive oil in a large skillet over medium heat. Add diced onion and minced garlic, and cook until softened, about 3-4 minutes.

2. Stir in curry powder and ground turmeric, and cook for another minute until fragrant.

3. Add diced tomatoes (including their juices) to the skillet, and simmer for 5 minutes.

4. Pour in coconut milk and bring the mixture to a gentle boil. Reduce heat to low and let it simmer for 10 minutes.

5. Stir in chickpeas and chopped spinach, and cook for an additional 5 minutes until heated through and spinach is wilted.

6. Season the chickpea and spinach curry with salt and pepper, and serve over cooked brown rice.

Nutritional Value (per serving): Calories: 380, Protein: 12g, Fat: 20g, Carbohydrates: 40g, Fiber: 10g

10. Eggplant and Tomato Caprese Salad (Serving Size: 1 plate)

Ingredients:
- 1 small eggplant, sliced into rounds
- 2 medium tomatoes, sliced
- 4 oz fresh mozzarella cheese, sliced
- ¼ cup fresh basil leaves
- 2 tablespoons balsamic vinegar
- 1 tablespoon olive oil
- Salt and pepper to taste

Instructions:
1. Preheat your grill or grill pan to medium-high heat. Brush eggplant slices with olive oil and season with salt and pepper.
2. Grill eggplant slices for 3-4 minutes on each side, until tender and lightly charred.
3. Arrange grilled eggplant, tomato slices, and fresh mozzarella cheese slices on a serving plate.
4. Drizzle balsamic vinegar over the top of the salad.
5. Garnish with fresh basil leaves before serving.

Nutritional Value (per serving): Calories: 280, Protein: 12g, Fat: 18g, Carbohydrates: 20g, Fiber: 8g

11. Spinach and Feta Stuffed Chicken Breast (Serving Size: 1 chicken breast)
Ingredients:
- 2 boneless, skinless chicken breasts
- 2 cups fresh spinach leaves
- ¼ cup crumbled feta cheese
- 2 cloves garlic, minced
- 1 tablespoon olive oil
- 1 teaspoon dried oregano

- Salt and pepper to taste

Instructions:
1. Preheat your oven to 375°F (190°C).
2. Using a sharp knife, cut a pocket horizontally into each chicken breast, being careful not to cut all the way through.
3. In a skillet, heat olive oil over medium heat. Add minced garlic and cook until fragrant, about 1 minute.
4. Add fresh spinach leaves to the skillet and cook until wilted, about 2-3 minutes. Remove from heat and let cool slightly.
5. Once cooled, mix wilted spinach with crumbled feta cheese. Stuff the spinach and feta mixture into the pockets of the chicken breasts.
6. Season the stuffed chicken breasts with dried oregano, salt, and pepper.
7. Place the stuffed chicken breasts in a baking dish and bake in the preheated oven for 25-30 minutes, or until chicken is cooked through and no longer pink in the center.

Nutritional Value (per serving): Calories: 320, Protein: 40g, Fat: 14g, Carbohydrates: 4g, Fiber: 2g

12. Quinoa and Vegetable Buddha Bowl (Serving Size: 1 bowl)

Ingredients:
- 1 cup cooked quinoa
- 1 cup mixed vegetables (roasted sweet potatoes, steamed broccoli, sautéed kale)
- ½ cup chickpeas, drained and rinsed
- ¼ avocado, sliced
- 2 tablespoons hummus
- 1 tablespoon tahini dressing
- Fresh lemon wedges, for serving
- Sesame seeds, for garnish

Instructions:
1. In a bowl, arrange cooked quinoa, mixed vegetables, and chickpeas.
2. Top with sliced avocado and dollops of hummus.
3. Drizzle tahini dressing over the Buddha bowl.
4. Garnish with sesame seeds and serve with fresh lemon wedges on the side.

Nutritional Value (per serving): Calories: 400, Protein: 18g, Fat: 15g, Carbohydrates: 50g, Fiber: 12g

13. Grilled Salmon with Asparagus

Ingredients:

- 2 salmon fillets (4-6 oz each)
- 1 bunch asparagus, trimmed
- 1 tablespoon olive oil
- 1 lemon, sliced
- Salt and pepper to taste
- Fresh dill for garnish

Instructions:
1. Preheat your grill to medium-high heat.
2. Rub the salmon fillets with olive oil and season with salt and pepper.
3. Place the salmon fillets and asparagus spears on the grill.
4. Grill salmon for 4-5 minutes per side, or until cooked through and flaky.
5. Grill asparagus for 3-4 minutes, or until tender-crisp.
6. Serve grilled salmon and asparagus with lemon slices and garnish with fresh dill.

Nutritional Value (per serving): Calories: 320, Protein: 30g, Fat: 20g, Carbohydrates: 6g, Fiber: 3g

14. Quinoa and Black Bean Salad
Ingredients:
- 1 cup cooked quinoa
- 1 can (15 oz) black beans, drained and rinsed

- 1 red bell pepper, diced
- 1 cup cherry tomatoes, halved
- ¼ cup chopped cilantro
- 1 avocado, diced
- 2 tablespoons lime juice
- 1 tablespoon olive oil
- Salt and pepper to taste

Instructions:
1. In a big bowl, combine cooked quinoa, black beans, diced red bell pepper, cherry tomatoes, and chopped cilantro.
2. Add diced avocado to the bowl and gently toss to combine.
3. In a small bowl, whisk together lime juice, olive oil, salt, and pepper to make the dressing.
4. Drizzle the dressing over the quinoa and black bean salad and toss to coat evenly.
5. Serve chilled or at room temperature.

Nutritional Value (per serving): Calories: 320, Protein: 10g, Fat: 15g, Carbohydrates: 40g, Fiber: 12g

15. Greek Chicken Gyro Bowl
Ingredients:
- 2 boneless, skinless chicken breasts
- 2 cups cooked brown rice

- 1 cup diced cucumber
- 1 cup cherry tomatoes, halved
- ½ cup crumbled feta cheese
- ¼ cup sliced red onion
- 2 tablespoons tzatziki sauce
- Fresh parsley for garnish

Instructions:
1. Season chicken breasts with salt and pepper, then grill or bake until cooked through.
2. Slice grilled chicken into strips.
3. In bowls, layer cooked brown rice, sliced grilled chicken, diced cucumber, cherry tomatoes, crumbled feta cheese, and sliced red onion.
4. Drizzle tzatziki sauce over the top of each bowl.
5. Garnish with fresh parsley before serving.

Nutritional Value (per serving): Calories: 380, Protein: 30g, Fat: 12g, Carbohydrates: 40g, Fiber: 6g

16. Mediterranean Stuffed Bell Peppers
Ingredients:
- 4 bell peppers, halved and seeds removed
- 1 cup cooked quinoa
- 1 can (15 oz) chickpeas, drained and rinsed

- 1 cup diced cucumber
- 1 cup cherry tomatoes, halved
- ½ cup crumbled feta cheese
- ¼ cup chopped kalamata olives
- 2 tablespoons olive oil
- 2 tablespoons lemon juice
- Salt and pepper to taste

Instructions:
1. Preheat your oven to 375°F (190°C).
2. In a big bowl, combine cooked quinoa, chickpeas, diced cucumber, cherry tomatoes, crumbled feta cheese, chopped kalamata olives, olive oil, lemon juice, salt, and pepper.
3. Stuff halved bell peppers with the quinoa mixture.
4. Place stuffed bell peppers in a baking dish and cover with foil.
5. Bake in the preheated oven for 25-30 minutes, or until peppers are tender.
6. Serve hot.

Nutritional Value (per serving): Calories: 280, Protein: 12g, Fat: 10g, Carbohydrates: 35g, Fiber: 8g

17. Spicy Shrimp and Zucchini Noodles
Ingredients:

- 8 oz shrimp, peeled and deveined
- 2 medium zucchini, spiralized into noodles
- 2 cloves garlic, minced
- 1 tablespoon olive oil
- 1 teaspoon red pepper flakes
- Salt and pepper to taste
- Fresh parsley for garnish

Instructions:

1. Heat olive oil in a large skillet over medium heat. Add minced garlic and red pepper flakes, and cook until fragrant.

2. Add shrimp to the skillet and cook until pink and opaque, about 2-3 minutes per side.

3. Add zucchini noodles to the skillet and toss with the shrimp and garlic mixture.

4. Cook for 2-3 minutes, until zucchini noodles are tender but still crisp.

5. Season with salt and pepper, and garnish with fresh parsley before serving.

Nutritional Value (per serving): Calories: 220, Protein: 25g, Fat: 8g, Carbohydrates: 10g, Fiber: 3g

18. Stuffed Portobello Mushrooms with Quinoa and Spinach

Ingredients:

- 4 large portobello mushrooms, stems removed
- 1 cup cooked quinoa
- 2 cups fresh spinach leaves
- ½ cup diced tomatoes
- ¼ cup grated Parmesan cheese
- 2 tablespoons balsamic glaze
- Salt and pepper to taste

Instructions:
1. Preheat your oven to 375°F (190°C).
2. Place portobello mushrooms on a baking sheet lined with parchment paper.
3. In a bowl, combine cooked quinoa, fresh spinach leaves, diced tomatoes, and grated Parmesan cheese.
4. Spoon quinoa mixture into the cavities of the portobello mushrooms.
5. Drizzle stuffed mushrooms with balsamic glaze.
6. Bake in the oven for 20-25 minutes, or until mushrooms are tender and filling is heated through.
7. Serve hot.

Nutritional Value (per serving): Calories: 180, Protein: 8g, Fat: 5g, Carbohydrates: 25g, Fiber: 5g

19. Tofu and Vegetable Stir-Fry

Ingredients:

- 8 oz firm tofu, pressed and cubed
- 2 cups mixed vegetables (such as bell peppers, broccoli, snap peas)
- 2 cloves garlic, minced
- 2 tablespoons soy sauce
- 1 tablespoon hoisin sauce
- 1 tablespoon sesame oil
- Cooked brown rice or quinoa for serving

Instructions:

1. Heat sesame oil in a large skillet or wok over medium-high heat. Add minced garlic and cook until fragrant.
2. Add cubed tofu to the skillet and cook until golden brown on all sides.
3. Add mixed vegetables to the skillet and stir-fry until tender-crisp.
4. In a small bowl, whisk together soy sauce and hoisin sauce. Pour sauce over the tofu and vegetables in the skillet.
5. Stir-fry for another 2-3 minutes, until everything is evenly coated in sauce.
6. Serve tofu and vegetable stir-fry hot over cooked brown rice or quinoa.

Nutritional Value (per serving): Calories: 250, Protein: 15g, Fat: 10g, Carbohydrates: 25g, Fiber: 5g

20. Lentil and Vegetable Soup

Ingredients:
- 1 cup dried green lentils, rinsed and drained
- 4 cups vegetable broth
- 1 onion, diced
- 2 carrots, diced
- 2 stalks celery, diced
- 2 cloves garlic, minced
- 1 teaspoon dried thyme
- Salt and pepper to taste
- Fresh parsley for garnish

Instructions:
1. In a large pot, combine dried green lentils, vegetable broth, diced onion, diced carrots, diced celery, minced garlic, dried thyme, salt, and pepper.
2. Bring the soup to a boil, then reduce heat and simmer for 25-30 minutes, or until lentils and vegetables are tender.
3. Adjust seasoning with additional salt and pepper if needed.
4. Serve hot, garnished with fresh parsley.

Nutritional Value (per serving): Calories: 220, Protein: 15g, Fat: 1g, Carbohydrates: 40g, Fiber: 15g

www.ingramcontent.com/pod-product-compliance
Lightning Source LLC
Chambersburg PA
CBHW050808260726

48660CB00004B/1310